The COMPLETE IDIOT'S GUIDE TO First Aid Basics

by Stephen J. Rosenberg, M.D.
and Karla Dougherty

alpha books

A Division of Macmillan General Reference
A Simon and Schuster Macmillan Company
1633 Broadway, New York, NY 10019-6785

#35651261

International Standard Book Number: 0-02-861099-7

Library of Congress Catalog Card Number: 95-083358

98 97 96   8 7 6 5 4 3 2 1

Interpretation of the printing code: the rightmost number of the first series of numbers is the year of the book's printing; the rightmost number of the second series of numbers is the number of the book's printing. For example, a printing code of 96-1 shows that the first printing occurred in 1996.

Printed in the United States of America.

This publication contains information based on the research and experience of its authors and is designed to provide useful advice with regard to the subject matter covered. The authors and publisher are not engaged in rendering medical or other professional services in this publication. Circumstances vary between patients and situations, and this publication is not intended to provide a basis for action in particular circumstances without consideration by a competent emergency or medical professional.

The authors and publisher expressly disclaim any responsibility for any liability, loss, or risk, personal or otherwise, which is incurred as a consequence, directly or indirectly, of the use and application of any of the contents of this book.

Publisher
Theresa Murtha

Development Editor
Lisa A. Bucki

Cover Designers
Dan Armstrong
Barb Kordesh

Illustrators
Ryan Oldfather
Jeff Yesh

Designer
Kim Scott

Production Team
Angela Calvert
Tricia Flodder
Erich J. Richter
Scott Tullis
Christy Wagner

Contents at a Glance

Contents

Foreword

Emergencies are in the news and on the television, from *RESCUE 911* (remember that number!) to *ER*. Do you wonder how you would cope if faced with a sudden medical emergency? You may well be the first person on the scene, and what you do can make a difference. This book is written for you.

Some of the things that make our lives richer leave us more exposed to illness and injury. Many of us are involved in fitness and sports activities. Others travel to remote areas for business or pleasure. We are at risk for disasters—natural or man-made, large or small—as we go about our daily lives. We live longer, but sometimes with chronic conditions that can become acute without warning. Each of the seasons of the year and of our lives has its own beauty, its own activities, and its own hazards.

People seem to have a natural urge to *do something* in a crisis. As an emergency room physician, I can tell you that the main thing you have to avoid is panic. *The Complete Idiot's Guide to First Aid Basics* will give you the information and techniques you need so that you will know what to do and how to do it. With this knowledge, you will have the confidence to remain calm. And when you are calm, your common sense can function. Your very presence will be reassuring to the victim and bystanders alike.

You will be pleased to learn that you can deal competently with a whole variety of problems. The first part of *The Complete Idiot's Guide to First Aid Basics* provides the most important how tos for recognizing and alleviating life-threatening emergencies. Review this part often. The second part provides simple and logical approaches to common problems, from animal bites to stomach aches, in alphabetical order. The last section addresses the particular problems of women, injuries from specific sports, and risks encountered while traveling. You need not be able to diagnose and cure all the problems listed, but if you can recognize them, you can offer simple, safe, and helpful care.

Medicine has become more complex and technically sophisticated over the years, but first aid is not just for the pros. This guide reminds the reader that a lot can be done with one's five senses and the contents of a first aid kit. It tells you what items belong in your kit, and it gives you step-by-step instructions for using them. The guide clarifies the priorities while providing first aid. You will learn to keep yourself safe, to prevent further harm to the victim, and to see that the most ugly or obvious injury is not always the most serious. You will become alert to the complications of common diseases. You will also learn to recognize the most urgent problems and to call for timely professional intervention (there's 911 again!). You will learn when a visit to your own physician the next day is advisable, and when you can provide definitive care.

Illness and injury are never convenient, but you can be more alert to the possibilities that are inherent in certain situations: a child who's allergic to bee stings, a toddler who puts everything in her mouth, a teen who has made the ball team, a relative who has a heart condition, the flu season, a heat wave, a cold snap, a day at the beach, a long trip. You can review the appropriate chapters and be ready to help. Remember, first aid really begins with prevention.

The authors of *The Complete Idiot's Guide to First Aid Basics* have written a well-designed and informative book. The special messages—the DOs and DON'Ts of first aid—are highlighted.

Karla Dougherty has, in addition to her other writings, previously collaborated on 14 books on medical topics. She presents the information in a style that is delightful to read, easy to comprehend, and organized to aid recall. She brings out the best in her coauthor.

Dr. Steven Rosenberg specializes in Rehabilitation Medicine. Who better to write a book about first aid than a physician who deals daily with the consequences of illness and injury? He also has an interest in Geriatric emergencies, a growing field that will likely affect us all.

They are to be commended for the vast amount of information this guide contains. Together, they have made the vocabulary of medical emergencies accessible. With clear writing and gentle humor, they teach the basics of first aid. As a bonus, you will better understand what the "pros" do on the scene or in the emergency room, on TV or in your lives.

Take this guide with you on vacation. Keep a copy in the bathroom with the first aid kit. Leave one out for the baby-sitter. Send it to college with the kids. Review it often. Each time, you will learn something new, interesting, and useful. Whether the victim is yourself, a loved one, or a stranger, the guide will help you provide effective and efficient first aid. As you apply the advice in this book, you will know the satisfaction of a job well done. You may deal with a small problem easily. You may recognize a vital emergency, stabilize the victim, and get appropriate help promptly. There are times you can do a lot, and times you cannot. There are times when you can intervene actively, and times when you must do the hard job of waiting. You can always strive to be calm, competent, and compassionate.

The Complete Idiot's Guide to First Aid Basics includes the guidance you need to provide first aid for many problems under many circumstances. It does so in a way that is easy to consult and remember. You might discover a special interest in first aid, take more courses, and even join an ambulance squad. Or you might just find yourself the first person on the scene of an emergency, and what you can do is save a life.

Jo-Ann L. Frank, M.D., FACEP
Katonah, NY

xix

Introduction

First aid is one of those things you want to know how to give—but never want to use. None of us wants to think of someone being hurt or injured in a sudden accident. None of us wants to think of someone in pain.

Unfortunately, life is filled with pain along with its joys. And there are times when you need to know what to do to deal with painful situations.

When your child cuts herself, when your spouse hurts his head, when a toddler falls into deep water, or when ants spoil the family picnic you need to use first aid skills. Those skills can make the difference between infection and health and, sometimes, between life and death.

Learning first aid isn't difficult. The most important thing is to not be afraid. A cool head, good instinct, and step-by-step information is all you need.

That's where this book comes in. *The Complete Idiot's Guide to First Aid Basics* is the only guide you'll ever need if someone nearby gets hurt. This book takes you from your medicine cabinet to first aid on the road. It provides a detailed description of everything from bruises to bandages, head injuries to heart attacks, snake bites to sprains. And along the way, you'll find tidbits, interesting facts, insights, and entertaining tips that will actually make this book fascinating to read—even when you don't need it!

In Part 1, "Emergencies Can't Wait," you'll learn the real basics of first aid care. You'll learn exactly what to do when seconds count—without missing a beat. You'll know when to treat, why to treat, and how to treat, and when it's best to wait for professional help. These "principles" will be invaluable when you need to give first aid.

Part 1 also includes a peek inside your medicine cabinet, providing a detailed list of what you need for a well-stocked "larder" that's ready to tackle any emergency. We've also described special items, because not all families are the same. There are special items you may need for children under 12, for teens, and households with older adults.

Finally, Part 1 offers the Top 10 "How Tos" of first aid. Like Letterman's famous lists (without the irreverence), they are countdowns of what you need to do in an emergency. You'll find how to take a pulse, perform mouth-to-mouth resuscitation, stop profuse bleeding, and make a sling, as well as six other key first aid techniques. We even include a special list of the new universal guidelines for safe and protective first aid care.

Part 2 is a much more specific section. In fact, it's most likely the one you'll refer to again and again. "Simple, Safe, Step-by-Step First Aid," is the complete A to Z low-down of the most common situations that require first aid. Simply look up the accident or problem and follow the instructions for treating it.

For example, let's say your child has been stung by a honeybee. You simply go to the Is (more specifically to "Insect Bites"), where you can read everything you need to know to ease your child's pain, remove the stinger, and watch for signs of possible allergic reaction.

As another example, if someone suffers a bad burn, you turn to the Bs, (more specifically, to "Bumps, Bruises, Burns, and Electric Shock"). Almost immediately, you'll be able to identify the severity of the burn and find how to treat it before infection sets in. You'll also learn what *not* to do, despite the medical myths that have been floating around for years. (No, butter is not spreadable when it comes to burns!)

Part 2 also covers how to deal with more serious ailments and mishaps, such as sudden heart attacks, drowning, and head injuries. These, too, are easy to find, and the instructions for help are easy to follow when those seconds count.

Because Part 2 is so complete, it's the longest section of this book—but it is by no means the only place to linger. Part 3, "First Aid for Women" is a special section that addresses situations specific to women's special needs. You'll find out how to treat common "come-and-go" afflictions such as breast tenderness, yeast infections, and PMS, as well as much more serious situations such as pregnancy emergencies. There's even a section for women who are about to go through or are currently going through menopause.

Part 4 covers your "leisure time" injuries and ailments. "Sports and Travel First Aid" is all about those accidents that occur just when you're having a fabulous time. The good news is that if you follow our instructions for injuries incurred during golf or tennis, soccer or swimming meets, camp outs, and trips abroad, you'll all soon be back on your feet—ready to continue your fun.

How to Make This Book Work for You

Reading this book *before* an emergency arises will enable you to be, as the scout motto says "prepared." Make this an "interactive" experience, in which you can learn and put into action, and to which you can refer anytime something happens. *The Complete Idiot's Guide to First Aid Basics* should be handy, right next to the traveling first aid kit, in the bathroom next to the cabinet, or on the night table next to the phone.

And, just to make it even easier to use, we've added brief highlights at the beginning of each chapter to give you a "preview" of what's in store so you won't waste any time. We've also added a section entitled "The Least You Need to Know" at the end of every chapter to summarize the most important facts you've just browsed through. After all, when seconds count, who has time to flip through endless pages? You want—and need—the information now!

Extras

No, we're not through yet. Just to ensure that you've received a complete—and entertaining education—we've added a series of shaded boxes throughout the box that highlight specific insights and precautions you'll need to thoroughly understand how to treat *any* first aid emergency.

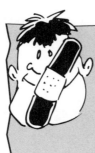

Before You Put the Band-Aid On

Boxes with this picture hold the "lighter side" of emergency first aid care. They provide those almost unknown facts that can make a difference, the truth behind medical myths that have been passed down through generations, and the insights that might make you pause (for only an instant) before you dig into that kit and come up with gauze.

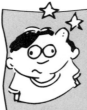

Ouch!

Look in boxes with this picture to find the important precautions you must take for a specific emergency. Read them. They can sometimes save a life!

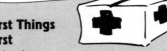

First Things First

This picture marks quick tips intended to facilitate first aid care and ensure safe treatment.

First Aids

Look to boxes with this picture to find definitions for medical words and descriptions you've always wanted to know but were perhaps too shy to ask about. This information will make the injuries and their treatments more understandable—and provide you with razor-sharp instincts.

Special Thanks

The Complete Idiot's Guide to First Aid Basics would not have been possible without the patients who have received Dr. Rosenberg's care: the ones that he saved and the ones for whom he did everything he could. A renowned expert in the field of neurology and geriatric emergencies, he knows, through experience and through his professorial lectures, from "whence he speaks."

Using his knowledge and expertise (and teaching capabilities), he taught me (Karla Dougherty, a medical writer), the ins and outs of first aid care. He made me understand the nuances, watch the signals, and work fast under conditions that are not exactly calm.

Both Dr. Rosenberg and myself want to thank Dr. Jo-Ann L. Frank, a doctor of Emergency Medicine for more than twenty years in upstate New York, for contributing her knowledge to the foreword of this book.

And it almost goes without saying that without the patience, expertise, and encouragement of our editors, Theresa Murtha and Lisa Bucki, this book would never have made it past the "idea" stage!

A special thank you also goes to our agent, Richard Parks, who has always stood by us during those "support needed" emergencies that, although not physical, are just as important to the creative mind.

Special Thanks from the Publisher to the Technical Reviewer

The Complete Idiot's Guide to First Aid Basics was reviewed by another physician, who double-checked the technical accuracy of what you'll learn here in order to help ensure that this book gives you everything you need to know to administer basic first aid. For that work, special thanks are extended to Dr. Jennifer J. Bucki.

A graduate of Indiana University School of Medicine, Jennifer J. Bucki, M.D., began working in the emergency department while a medical student. Her training in internal medicine included emergency medicine rotations as well as "walk-up clinic" experience. During a missionary trip to South America, she provided basic medical care to native populations in isolated regions on the continent. While an undergraduate zoology major at Butler University in Indianapolis, Indiana, she enjoyed classes such as tropical field biology and entomology in addition to her pre-med studies. She is certified by the American Board of Internal Medicine and is currently affiliated with one of the largest hospitals in the Midwest.

Trademarks

All terms mentioned in this book that are known to be or are suspected of being trademarks or service marks have been appropriately capitalized. Alpha Books and Macmillan General Reference cannot attest to the accuracy of this information. Use of a term in this book should not be regarded as affecting the validity of any trademark or service mark.

One More Word (Okay, a Few More Words) Before We Begin...

In short, this book is jam-packed with everything you need to know for emergencies. We're glad you have it in hand and, although this might sound odd, we hope you'll never have to use it!

The nineteenth century philosopher Charles Edward Montague once reported, "A gifted small girl has explained that pins are a great means of saving life, 'by not swallowing them.'"

However, thanks to this complete, thorough, and easy-to-use first aid guide, if someone did happen to eat a handful of pins, you'd know what to do!

Here's to health and successful first aid!

Part 1
Emergencies Can't Wait

You never know when someone you love—or even a stranger walking next to you on the street—may suddenly fall ill, break a leg, step out in front of a speeding car, or …well, you get the picture.

When someone you love gets hurt, it puts things in perspective. Suddenly, you stop thinking about those bills that need to be paid, the shopping you have to do for dinner, the deadline you have to meet at work. Life-threatening injuries are a real emergency. And when someone gets hurt, that emergency takes precedence over everything else in the entire world.

This book is about the emergencies that get in the way of good health despite our best intentions. And this particular part gets you off to a racing start (speed is essential in an emergency), providing you with first aid basics ranging from what items you should include in the "perfect" first aid kit to how to check for vital life signs, and from handling panic to treating a bleeding wound until help comes.

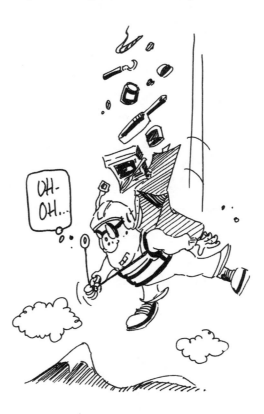

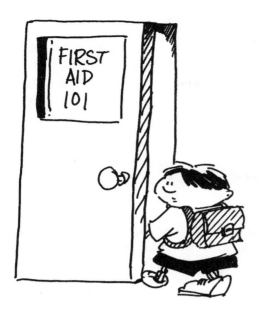

First Aid 101

Boom! It happened. An accident. Maybe it happened on vacation. Maybe it was at the family picnic. Maybe it was on a quiet night during the week. Whatever the case, accidents do happen, and knowing at least the rudimentary rules of first aid can make a difference. You can help when seconds—not minutes—count.

Here you'll find the important basic principles you need to know to improve your reaction time, your efficiency, and your ability to handle emergency situations. With these basics under your belt, you can be confident that your instincts are right. In later chapters, you'll find step-by-step instructions for actually beginning emergency procedures in those first few crucial moments. The combination of these basic principles and those instructions will help you take charge fast—and possibly save a life.

Principle 1: Use the Tools You Have

The words "first aid" probably conjure up visions of Band-Aids, ice compresses, and Ace bandages. In actuality, the most immediate and necessary tools for dealing with health emergencies aren't found in a kit or a cabinet. They are found on your person. They *are* your person—more specifically, your hands, your ears, your eyes, and your instincts.

Instincts are one thing, but don't underestimate the power of observation. When an experienced physician uses his or her gut reaction to make a diagnosis, it isn't just an instinctive feeling. To make a good, quick diagnosis, he also uses his eyes, ears, nose, and sense of touch. The clue is to know what to be watching for, and a good physician goes "right to the punch." Is the victim breathing? What does the breathing sound like? Are the eyes focused? Are there bruises and bumps on the body? What's the victim's reaction time when touched or spoken to? Combine your instincts with your powers of observation, and you'll have an unbeatable combination to help save a life!

Principle 2: Don't Panic!

It's easy to say "Don't panic," but if someone you love is injured, that's often difficult to do. If someone is unconscious, bleeding, crying, or hysterical, even the most calm "first aider" can panic.

Just remember: You'll be able to help the person much more if you remain calm and think through a situation. First, take a deep breath and count to three. Disassociate yourself from the situation. The important thing is to remain calm. You can panic later—when trained help finally arrives.

Principle 3: Determine Whether to Treat—or Wait

It's often easy to see the injuries that need immediate attention. You can usually identify and begin to treat profuse bleeding, respiratory distress, sprained arms and legs, and cardiac arrest using only your eyes and ears. (See Chapters 3 and 4 for such key first aid treatments as making splints, making bandages, and performing mouth-to-mouth resuscitation.) But some conditions are not so obvious. Unconsciousness, for example, can be a sign of shock or head injury—both of which can be very serious. Unfortunately, these can't be treated with direct pressure or mouth-to-mouth. In fact, the best thing to do is cover the person with a blanket and get help fast. (See Part 2 for treating specific injuries ranging from choking to head injury, animal bites to splinters—all arranged alphabetically.)

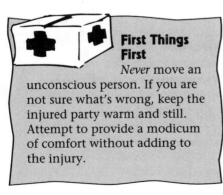

First Things First

Never move an unconscious person. If you are not sure what's wrong, keep the injured party warm and still. Attempt to provide a modicum of comfort without adding to the injury.

Principle 4: Keep a List of Emergency Phone Numbers

It's a good feeling to be prepared. Whether you simply reach for your cellular, run a half a block to the nearest phone, or pick up the extension in the kitchen, it's nice to know you'll know exactly who to call. In addition to 911, every home should have an easily accessible list of emergency phone numbers that includes police, fire and ambulance, and poison control. If possible, program them into your phones for speed-dialing in an emergency.

Principle 5: Remember Your ABCs

Checking for vital signs of life is obviously a priority in first aid care. That's why you'll notice we talk a lot about checking pulses, listening for breathing, and recognizing signs of shock. (Chapters 3 and 4 cover first aid treatment in the event of weak vital signs or no vital signs.)

To help you remember which vital signs to check, remember your ABCs. These ABCs have nothing to do with reading and writing, but if you can think of them in the correct order, you *might* save a life.

➤ Airways Open. Look: Be sure to see if a person is breathing. Watch for steady intakes of breath and exhalations. Listen: Can you hear breathing? Is the breathing ragged or uneven? Help keep airways clear and accessible by placing one hand under an injured person's neck and gently tilting his or head back to keep the mouth and nose unobstructed.

➤ Breathing Restored. An unconscious person will breath better if he or she is on her back in a prone position. A conscious person will do better either sitting up or semi-reclining. Keep clothing around the neck and shoulders loose. Reassure the injured person, calming him or her in an attempt to prevent emotional breathing problems such as anxiety-induced hyperventilation.

If an injured person is awake, try to find out if he or she has any history of heart disease. Shortness of breath can be a symptom of cardiac distress (which is covered in detail in Chapter 17).

Ouch!
Even if the environment is safe or if you think a person might have hurt his or her head or back, you might have to consider moving the person. For example, if you cannot detect breathing, if you are not getting a pulse, or if you are nowhere near emergency help, you might not have a choice. Hopefully, your car, your boat, or your *arms* are in good working order!

If you detect shallow breathing or no breathing, make sure nothing is clogging passageways by hooking your fingers and checking a person's throat. Perform mouth-to-mouth resuscitation (see Chapter 3) if the person doesn't appear to be breathing. Get help as fast as you can!

➤ Circulation Maintained. Checking for a pulse is as crucial as making sure the victim can breathe. The heart, after all, must send blood oxygen to the lungs for breath (and to the brain for this basic instruction). Take the injured person's pulse (as you'll learn in Chapter 3). If you can't find a pulse, begin CPR *if* you are trained and certified to do so. If not, do mouth-to-mouth resuscitation (see Chapter 3) and scream for help.

It might sound obvious, but the best way to determine if a person is unconscious or awake is to shout in his or her ear. If you get no response, you know he or she is out—and you don't have to count to ten.

Principle 6: Avoiding Infection for Yourself and the Injured Person

In today's world, where HIV (the virus that causes AIDS) and other infections abound, universal safety guidelines are imperative in any situation. This principal pinpoints the necessary (and simple) precautions you'll need to know to protect yourself against any infection or disease an injured person might have. Because most deadly viruses, such as HIV, are spread through contact of bodily fluids (blood, saliva, and substances that have been vomited up), these universal guidelines are crucial for both you and the victim.

The following illustration shows a number of items that can protect you from infection and disease. As you'll learn in the following sections, you should keep an airway bag, disposable gloves, and heavy duty protective bags (for disposal of infectious or hazardous waste) in your first aid kit.

Wash Your Hands

There's a reason why doctors "scrub up" before an operation. You won't have the luxury of a germ-free environment if you find yourself administering first aid in an emergency, but there are a few things you can do to protect yourself.

Wash your hands with hot water and soap if possible. However, in case you're nowhere near a sink (or even a river bed), keep a few "wet naps" in your first aid kid. Cleanse your hands with them. If worse comes to worse, you can even use the alcohol or antibacterial lotion you'll be using to clean a wound.

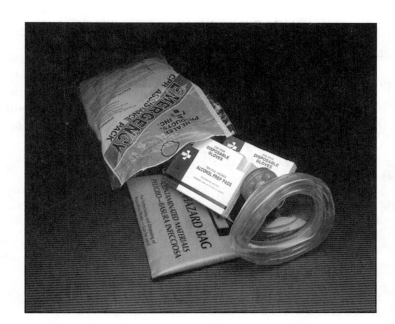

Universal safety devices prevent the spread of germs and infection.

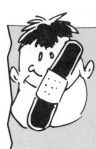

Before You Put the Band-Aid On

Here's a natural germ fighter: the ocean. The salt in the water helps wash away germs and keep infections at bay. You might not be able to take a sip if you're thirsty, but if you need to wash your hands, you might not have to look further than the horizon!

Wear Gloves

It's a good idea to keep a couple pair of disposable latex gloves in your first aid kit. When you're treating an open wound, gloves can protect you from most contagions. You can purchase latex gloves from a hardware store or medical supply store. If you can't seem to locate any in your neighborhood, simply ask your dentist or physician where they purchase their gloves the next time you're in the office! You might also want to ask them about prices, too.

Wear a Gown, Apron, or Cover-Up

Obviously, if you're in the midst of a life-or-death situation, you're not going to have those "George Clooney-ER-greens" at hand. But use common sense—especially if a person is bleeding. If you've been in the water, cover up over your swimsuit and bare skin. If

7

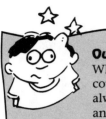

Ouch!
When seconds count, there isn't always time to get an airway bag from your first aid kit (which might be in the car, parked 200 yards away). Although airway bags are best, you *can* perform mouth-to-mouth resuscitation in a safe fashion without them. You can use salt water, alcohol, or even soda poured on a cloth or a piece of clothing to wash the victim's mouth and nose. If the person is bleeding around the mouth or nose, use a handkerchief or other lightweight, porous cloth to keep the blood away from you as you work.

you're wearing an open jacket, zip it up. You're better to be safe and cover up unless seconds literally count.

And, while you're tying on your gown, don't forget the dental dam. A cross between a football player's mouth gear and a molar mold, this device protects your mouth from any fluids that can accidentally squirt up and in.

Use Disposable Airway Bags

Airway bags let you perform mouth-to-mouth resuscitation without making contact between with the other person's mouth. These handy gadgets can be found in many prepackaged first aid kits today. Basically, an airway bag places a barrier between your mouth and the injured person's mouth to prevent the spread of disease.

Use Protective Glasses

Glasses or any type of goggles help protect your eyes from possible splashing from an open wound. If sunglasses are all you have available, you might be safer if you have them on—even if it's dark outside.

Be Aware of Sharp Objects

If you have to treat a puncture wound caused by an arrow, knife, fishing hook, or rusty nail, apply antibacterial ointments and antiseptics around the wound. Never try to remove a large object; sometimes the only thing preventing profuse bleeding is the object in the hole! See Chapter 24 for specific instructions on when to remove a foreign object and when to leave it alone. And don't forget to wear your protective gear, just in case a puncture wound opens up further or the sharp object accidentally slashes you.

Get help as fast as you can. Clean the wound, and then make the injured person as comfortable as you can while you wait for help to arrive. And one final precaution: Don't take off your gloves or your other protective gear until you're near a hot shower and soap far from the scene.

Use a Mask

Handkerchiefs make great masks. (Just ask any cowboy with a bandanna around his neck who's ever been caught in a dust storm.) To avoid possible airborne contagions, especially if you are helping a stranger whose medical history you do not know, simply tie a handkerchief or scarf around your mouth and nose. (Of course, if you have to do mouth-to-mouth resuscitation, you'll have to remove the mask!)

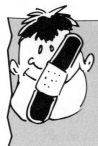

Before You Put the Band-Aid On

Fourteen states have passed a "Good Smaritan Law," which provides legal protection for persons who administer emergency first aid. In other words, if you try to help someone to the best of your ability, you can not be found guilty of negligence. Let the good works begin!

Principle 7: Know What to Do (A Top 10 List)

Obviously, you need to know what to do before you can start anything, especially when it comes to a life or death emergency. The best advice? Browse through this book—especially all of Part 1. You'll give your instincts and your powers of observation an important exercise in emergency first aid. To avoid forgetting everything you've learned, here are the rules of first aid emergency care in nutshell. If time's a'wastin', don't worry. Just look over this Top 10 checklist, and you'll be prepared to begin your first aid care for real!

1. **Shout for help!** Don't be afraid to use your lungs and shout for help as soon as you begin first aid measures. Keep shouting for help until you know you've been heard and action has been taken. Professional help can't come soon enough—if it's needed!

2. **Assess the situation and scout the territory.** If possible, ask the injured person what happened. Can she speak? Can she tell you how serious the accident is? Also, look around and make sure that performing first aid isn't going to be hazardous to *your* health. Are there any exposed wires near the injured person? Are there toxic fumes or flames? Is the ice hard enough for you to walk on or the water calm enough to jump in? In short, make sure you aren't in any danger before you start first aid. You won't be much help if you get injured, too.

3. **Determine if the accident warrants a visit to a hospital—or simply a cleansing and a Band-Aid.** If the injured person can talk, great. If the person simply needs stitches, don't call for an ambulance, just make a trip to the emergency room. But if he or she is unconscious, you need to make that 911 call. Check those important ABCs: Are the airways clear? Is he or she breathing? What about circulation? Is there a pulse? And, most importantly, it's up to you to decide whether or not to move the injured person. Sometimes this can't be helped. Once you've decided that you can

safely walk on the ice or run past the flames, you might have to save the person in jeopardy by pulling or carrying them to safety, away from flames, thin ice, or toxic fumes. Here's a good rule to remember: don't move a person if there isn't a life-or-death reason to do so. You might cause more harm than good.

4. **If you are trained and certified in CPR and a person is choking or cannot breathe, begin CPR right away.** If you are not trained in CPR, do *not* attempt to resuscitate. You can break the ribs or puncture the lungs, for example, and if the person is choking, you can actually force the object further down his or her throat! If you don't know CPR, use mouth-to-mouth resuscitation techniques (see Chapter 3) or for choking, use the Heimlich Maneuver (see Chapter 9). Also, take the injured person's pulse and loosen his or her clothes to make breathing easier.

5. **Stop the bleeding.** If the injured person is bleeding, apply direct, even pressure with a cloth and your hands to slow the flow. (To protect yourself against HIV and other infections while in direct contact with blood, don't forget to practice the universal guidelines for preventing infection, covered in detail at the end of this chapter.) Lift up a bleeding limb if it doesn't cause substantial additional pain. Make and apply a tourniquet only as a last resort. (See "How to Stop Bleeding" in Chapter 3 for details on using a tourniquet.)

6. **Treat any symptoms of shock.** If the victim is chilled, breathing harshly, nauseous, clammy, and pale, it is possible he or she is in shock and might become unconscious at any time. (See Chapter 3 for treating shock.) Vomiting can also be a sign of shock, and you want to keep airways clear. If no back or neck injury is suspected, gently roll your the victim's whole body to the side to keep airways open and prevent vomit from pooling in the back of the throat (which can cause choking). Cover the victim with a blanket if you see any signs of shock. Use the universal guidelines to prevent transmittal of HIV or any other infection (covered later in this chapter) if you come in contact with bodily fluids.

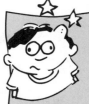

Ouch!
Don't move an injured person if you don't have to. As long as you're not in a burning building or drowning at sea, it is best to let a person lie where he or she is. If the victim has back, head, or neck injuries, moving him or her can make the injuries worse or even cause permanent damage or death.

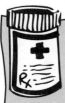

First Aids
CPR is short for Cardiopulmonary Resuscitation. When administered immediately to a patient suffering cardiac or respiratory distress, CPR can save a life. However, it's best to take a course to learn CPR. It's not safe to rely solely on the knowledge you gain from reading a book. You need to be certified in order to perform CPR correctly and save lives.

7. **Look for a Medic Alert bracelet or necklace.** The medic alert identification tag (shown in the following figure) bears the name "Medic Alert" and displays the Greek symbol for medical care (a snake twisted around a staff). This bracelet provides medical and emergency personnel with life-sustaining information about the patient's medical history and special needs. The Medic Alert tag tells you if the victim is diabetic, epileptic, or allergic to any medications—all of which can make a tremendous difference in the course of treatment. If there is no Medic Alert bracelet or necklace, check the injured person's wallet. Sometimes medical warnings are written on an ID card or driver's license.

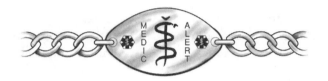

Look for a Medic Alert medallion like this on either a necklace or bracelet.

8. **Seek trained medical assistance.** At this point, you can leave the injured person for a moment if necessary to summon help. In this world of cellular phones, it's nice to know we're only an arm's length away from 911. But what if an injury takes place where there isn't a portable phone? Or what if you don't own one yourself? Shout for help or as a last resort, run to the nearest phone. When you call for help, tell the police you want an ambulance with an EMT staff. Only trained personnel can help you with cardiac or respiratory problems, head traumas, poisoning, or fractures.

   With or without medical alert information, you can make your call to 911 more efficient if you begin with your name and location and the nature of the problem. If you've performed steps 1 through 7, you can also inform them of such additional things as potential dangers in the locale, whether or not the patient is breathing or bleeding or appears to have broken bones. All of these things help the EMTs prepare themselves before they arrive on the scene.

9. **Never give an injured unconscious person anything by mouth.** This means no pills, no liquids—nothing! When a person is unconscious, even water (which you might think will ease the pain) can interfere with breathing and choke him or her.

10. **Wait.** This is the hardest part of administering first aid care. When you've followed the steps above and done everything you can, all that's left is to wait for the ambulance to arrive. Unfortunately, minutes can feel like hours. While you're waiting, try to keep the injured person calm. You can provide comfort with a soothing voice or a gentle touch. The "Ssh. Don't worry. Help is almost here..." will help you cope as much as it will help the person you're treating.

The Least You Need to Know

➤ Don't panic! Take a deep breath and check for vital signs (breathing and pulse) while you call for help.

➤ Loosen the injured person's clothing, and drape a warm blanket around him or her to treat symptoms of shock.

➤ Do not move an injured person unless it is unavoidable. Doing so could cause or worsen head, neck, or back injuries.

➤ Staunch any bleeding by applying pressure (see Chapter 3 for more information).

➤ Be prepared. If you're away from home, pull out your cellular phone if you have one and dial 911. Otherwise, run to the closest public phone, shouting for help all the way. And keep a list of emergency phone numbers by your telephone at home.

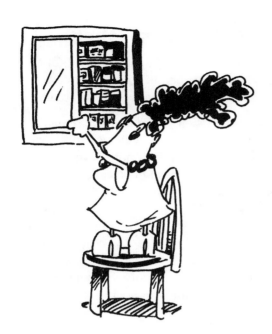

Chapter 2

The Home Medicine Cabinet

In This Chapter

➤ An easy and inexpensive home first aid kit

➤ Special needs for children and teens

➤ What every effective first aid kit must contain

Picture this: Your curious toddler, ready to touch and examine anything he sees, stumbles over a chair en route to the doggie's dish. The chair falls. His knee is cut and bleeding profusely. You've read this book and you know one of the first basic principles of first aid care: don't panic. You also know you need to stop the bleeding. With words of comfort, you quickly reach for the emergency kit you keep in the kitchen on the top shelf. It's all ready to use, complete with a list of emergency phone numbers pasted to the inside of the top.

As it turns out, your child's bleeding looked worse than it really was. A little antiseptic ointment and a sturdy bandage, and he's okay. It's one thing to know the first steps to take in a medical emergency, but it's quite another to have the supplies at hand. This chapter outlines the basic materials you would need to administer first aid in the event of an emergency. By the way, don't forget where you keep your first aid kit!

The 21 First Aid Items Every Home Should Have

The following items are necessities for any first aid kit. Prepackaged kits are great for the road. You can buy inexpensive "all-purpose" kits to keep in each of your cars and in almost every room of your house! See Chapter 34 for the best prepackaged kits around.

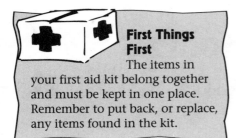

First Things First
The items in your first aid kit belong together and must be kept in one place. Remember to put back, or replace, any items found in the kit.

But space is not an issue when you're living at home. You can have the luxury of filling your medicine cabinet with everything you might need—in the amounts you want. You don't need the convenience of prepackaged first aid kits. You can buy all the items you need in a drugstore or supermarket. You can either keep them in a medicine cabinet or in a childproof container that's readily available in a kitchen cabinet or a closet. Be sure to store it where anyone can locate it quickly, and make sure everyone knows where it is! And, no matter what type of kit you have, make sure you place a list of emergency phone numbers inside the lid. Include numbers for your doctor, the local hospital, poison control center, and more.

In order to have a useful first aid kit, you will need to purchase the following items:

1. *Protective gear to prevent the spread of infection.* Remember those universal guidelines? Chances are, if an accident occurs within your intimate family, you won't have to bother with gloves, goggles, aprons, and dental dams. But it's useful to have these items in your medicine cabinet just in case someone other than your intimate family has an accident in your home. And it's a good idea to put protective gear (especially latex gloves, disposable airway bags, goggles or masks, and dental dams) in your traveling kits or to add them to your prepackaged kits. It's especially important to practice safety measures if you happen to help a stranger. You don't want to transmit HIV or any other virus or disease from one person to another.

2. *Adhesive bandages* in an assortment of sizes for any punctures, cuts, or minor scrapes. Be sure to buy bandages that are sterile and come individually wrapped.

3. *Sterile gauze pads* that are individually wrapped may be useful for larger cuts, profuse bleeding, burns, and infections.

4. *A roll of adhesive surgical tape* will come in handy when using gauze pads. You will need the tape to secure the cotton pad to the laceration. First aid adhesive tape is great for wounds that need to be sealed from infection. This tape is extremely sticky, anyone who has ever yanked off a taped bandage knows that it can be a painful experience. Clear tape will stretch with the body; it is especially effective when waterproofing is necessary. Paper tape is best for individuals with sensitive skin, or if the dressings need to be frequently changed. If you want a recommendation, use *cloth tape*. It keeps a gauze bandage secured without the irritation or discomfort of the other adhesive tapes.

5. *Scissors* may be necessary to cut tape, clothing, or bandages in emergency situations. Surgical scissors will cut tape cleanly and quickly, but any good scissors will do in an emergency. (Avoid "kiddie scissors" if possible; they're meant for cutting out paper dolls and designs.)

6. *Elastic bandages*, or Ace bandages (the common brand name), with clips may be used for sprains and twists.

7. *Sterile cotton balls* for applying ointments and antiseptics, as well as a sterile cloth for washing and dressing cuts and abrasions

8. *Tweezers* for removing any foreign objects from a cut or for splinters. Although needles are only good for splinters, they can sometimes get out a small foreign object better. So keep one on hand in your first aid cabinet.

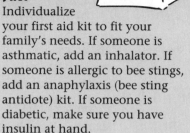

First Things First

Individualize your first aid kit to fit your family's needs. If someone is asthmatic, add an inhalator. If someone is allergic to bee stings, add an anaphylaxis (bee sting antidote) kit. If someone is diabetic, make sure you have insulin at hand.

Before You Put the Band-Aid On

Sterile and *germ-free* are crucial words when finding supplies to treat wounds. The sterile products need to be used in order to avoid infection. Bandages and cotton balls are purchased sterile. But when using your own medical "tools," you must be able to sterilize them after each use. You can do this by lighting a match and moving the instrument back and forth through the flame. Just don't forget to add a pack of matches to your first aid kit! Alcohol and peroxide can also be used for sterilization.

9. *Matches* can be a useful addition to your medicine cabinet's first aid section. In an emergency, a flame will sterilize needles and tweezers. Just make sure you keep the pack out of the reach of tiny curious hands!

10. *Rubbing alcohol* can be used to clean utensils in your first aid kit, and it very effectively cleans cuts, scrapes, and minor wounds. Antibacterial antiseptic lotions and ointments should be added to your homemade kit as well. Bacitracin or Johnson's & Johnson's First Aid Cream are

First Aids

Histamines are chemicals produced by mast cells—fat, chubby cells that are found in our skin. These chemicals are inflammatory, causing itching and burning. *Antihistamine* medications actually neutralize the histamines in the mast cells, which stops the itching.

good all-around ointments that will prevent infections on scraped knees, cuts, and wounds. They also make excellent dressings.

11. *Oral and rectal thermometers* are important (and petroleum jelly for the rectal thermometer). Fever can be a sign of shock, poisoning, or infection. It's always good to gauge a sick person's temperature to know how to proceed. (See Part 2 for specific sections on fever and poisoning; see Chapter 3 for treating shock and stopping infection in its tracks.)

12. *Calamine lotion* for insect bites and hives. This lotion is used to relieve itching and scratching. It also contains a healing agent which is especially useful for poison ivy.

13. *Antihistamine tablets* are good to have handy in case of an allergic reaction, an attack of the sneezes and sniffles, a sinus problem, or a migraine headache (all signs of allergic reactions to pollen or dust). Benadryl is a good antihistamine, and it even comes in a cream to treat superficial allergic reactions, such as rashes and hives.

14. *Mineral oil and Q-tips* to remove ticks on the skin and foreign objects from ears. Simply dab a little oil on the Q-tip and gently touch the area in question.

15. *Sterile eye wash* for eye injuries.

16. *Syrup of Ipecac*, which will induce vomiting in case of poisoning. Available in any drugstore, Syrup of Ipecac's sole purpose is for inducing the vomiting reflex. The syrup is made from a South American root and does not require a prescription to purchase. Only use Syrup of Ipecac if you know exactly what an injured person swallowed. Vomiting can worsen symptoms of some poisons, such as petroleum and corrosive chemical products. To be absolutely certain whether to induce vomiting or not, call your local poison center immediately.

17. *A bar of soap* or a container of antibacterial liquid soap to clean wounds and your own hands. Sealed "wet naps" also work well.

18. *An ice pack* to reduce swelling, to cool a victim, or to reduce fever. (Many companies now make "instant" ice packs that do not need to be chilled. Chemicals keep them cold so you can store them in a first aid kit.)

19. *A flashlight.* Be sure to check the flashlight batteries frequently. Flares need to be kept in the car or boat to alert passers-by of an emergency condition. Flares not only prevent unforeseen collisions in the dark, they force other drivers to slow down (and someone might just offer help or the emergency phone call you desperately need).

20. *Medicine for diarrhea* such as Pepto-Bismol, Immodium AD, or Mylanta.

21. *Aspirin, acetaminophen (Tylenol), or ibuprofen (Advil)* tablets to relieve pain and reduce fever. Remember that some people are allergic to aspirin, and some have bleeding or stomach problems that aspirin can make worse. When in doubt, opt for the Tylenol or Advil. NEVER give aspirin for a fever to children under 18 years of age; they are particularly susceptible to Reye's syndrome, a form of brain damage that can occur when aspirin is taken for a fever. Instead, give your kids Tylenol for Children, or Pediaprofen (a child's version of ibuprofen). Ditto for pregnant moms!

22. *Large, triangular pieces of cloth* (scarves) for makeshift slings, splints, and tourniquets.

Special Items for Children Under Twelve

Remember that trip your whole family took to Williamsburg—when your youngest child suddenly got the worst cold of her life? The fact is that young kids tend to experience sudden illnesses more often than their older siblings or their parents. Further, young kids need different doses of medication and treatment. They can take the same medications and ointments as their older counterparts, but NOT AS MUCH. In short, read the labels of your pain relievers, your cough syrups, and your creams before you use them for your children. Even better, check out your drugstore shelf and put a supply of baby aspirin and other specific children's medications in your first aid kit. And don't forget to pack that baby aspirin, Tylenol, or Pediaprofen for those "on-the-road" emergencies! Maybe—just maybe—you'll get to enjoy your vacation after all!

Special items for kids that you need to pack in your first aid kit include:

1. Baby aspirin but only for aches, pains, and strains. Kids under 18 years old with fevers should only take Tylenol for Children or Pediaprofen (a child's version of Advil) to avoid the risk of Reye's Syndrome, a dangerous ailment that affects the nervous system.

2. Warm blankets.

3. A small stuffed animal.

4. Towels to use as makeshift pillows, immobilizing equipment for head and back injuries, or simply to wipe up dirt, sweat, and vomit.

5. Baby powder to add a soothing touch.

6. Children's cough syrup.

7. A music box or favorite cassette and walkman for distraction.

8. Adhesive tape with "fun" designs and shapes.

9. Cloth tape (it's easier to remove).

10. A bright bandanna for use as a sling or splint (anything to help distract the child).

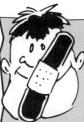

Before You Put the Band-Aid On

Small kids like to put things in their mouths. The trouble starts when they swallow something like a coin or a twig. If that happens, first look in the child's mouth; it's possible that the object is not wedged too far down and you can pull it out with sterile tweezers. If the child is definitely choking, begin the Heimlich Maneuver. (See Chapter 9 for special Heimlich Maneuver techniques for children.)

The Top Teen List

Administering first aid care to teenagers is not too different from administering it to children. If anything, teens can be more fearful because they are more aware of what's going on. A child might feel pain in her arm, but a teen will know she's broken it. If a child can't move, it will be scary, but a soothing word and touch can go far. This is not so with teens. If a teen can't move, he or she will be terrified. The last thing many teens want is to be touched by an "adult." Panic must be avoided at all costs. If soothing words don't help, explain calmly what you are doing and why. Have the teen become a part of your "first aid treatment team." It's a good distraction until help comes.

Teens can handle most adult medications, but there are a few extra items that can help when a teenager is injured:

1. A warm blanket.

2. Pad and pencil. (If a teen can't talk, he can write answers to your questions. This is a good distraction device.)

3. A walkman and a few favorite cassettes for distraction.

4. Non-alcoholic cough medicine.

5. Buffered aspirin or acetaminophen (Tylenol), which are easier on nervous stomachs.

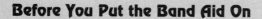

Before You Put the Band Aid On

Statistics show that teenagers are the ones most likely to "experiment" with drug and alcohol abuse. It's best to administer the following treatment for a possible drug overdose.

Make sure the teen is lying prone, on his or her back. Loosen clothing and place a warm blanket around him or her. Talk to the victim, and then talk some more. A calm, soothing voice will help place the teen in reality if he or she is hysterical.

Adult First Aid Supplies

The list of items every home should have (presented early in this chapter) covers what you will need for adult first aid emergencies. It doesn't hurt to have a comforting voice and a soothing touch when dealing with young adults and children. And a warm blanket and some warm words won't hurt an adult in pain either! Here are some extras you might want to keep on hand specifically for adults:

1. Anaphylaxis kits are essential if any family member is allergic to bee stings. This simple antidote will reduce the inflammation and swelling in the airways and help the victim breathe again!

2. Nitroglycerin tablets are good to have on hand if anyone in your family has a history of heart pain or angina.

3. Inhalers are necessary for anyone who has asthma. Keep several on hand in case it takes a while for help to arrive.

4. Irritated eyes? Make sure you have eye drops to soothe allergic irritation, as well as eye washes to help cleanse eyes of any chemicals that might have accidentally gotten in the eyes. (See Chapter 11 for specific eye first aid.)

5. Ear drops will help reduce earaches caused by infections and fevers. They will also help remove an overload of wax or a stubborn insect, and they can help restore inner ear equilibrium.

6. You don't need to keep a vial of glucose on hand, but if someone feels a sudden drop in the middle of the afternoon, it could be a low blood sugar reaction. The solution? Keep a few packets of sugar on hand to place on the tongue. Give the person a slice of protein (low-fat cheese or turkey is healthy) and a slice of bread to stabilize blood sugar levels.

7. Insulin tablets or injections are imperative in an any first aid kit if someone you know has diabetes.

8. Contrary to popular opinion, a "nip" of brandy is not good medicine. It doesn't really keep you warmer or help you stay calm. (And, remember, in Chapter 1, we advised never to give a person in trouble anything to drink!) However, if you are the one performing the first aid, that brandy might taste mighty good after the crisis.

9. A warm blanket or one of those new shiny, lightweight insulated covers (used by astronauts in space) will help keep your loved one warm. Keep a warm blanket in the trunk of your car or within reach on a shelf in the closet.

10. A plain brown "lunch bag" can be used to ward off panic attacks. Simply have the victim breathe into a bag for several minutes to help steady breathing. It's also a good idea to have a supply of anti-anxiety medication on hand if anyone in your family has a history of anxiety or panic attacks.

The Least You Need to Know

➤ A well-stocked medicine cabinet or first aid kit has, at the very least, aspirin, adhesive tape, a thermometer, sterile gauze bandages, tape, tweezers, anti-diarrhea medicine, rubbing alcohol, and an antibiotic cream.

➤ Keep a blanket and a (working) flashlight on hand.

➤ Read the labels. Make sure children and young teens are given correct dosages.

➤ Never forget the power of a soothing touch and a calm voice. It can help an injured person of any age.

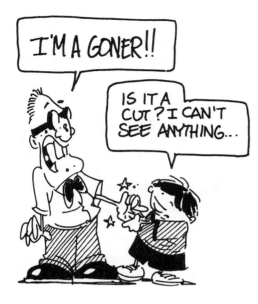

Chapter 3

Vital Emergencies: The First Top Five "How Tos"

In This Chapter

➤ Taking a pulse and finding a heartbeat

➤ Stopping the bleeding and dressing cuts

➤ Watching for infection

➤ Performing mouth-to-mouth resuscitation effectively

➤ Recognizing the signs of shock

Take the injured victim's pulse. If there seem to be broken bones, make a sling. Stop the bleeding by applying pressure. Perform mouth-to-mouth resuscitation. We all know what these commands mean, but what about actually performing the actions they describe? Can you effectively find a pulse? Can you make a sling? And, if someone isn't breathing, do you know the first thing about mouth-to-mouth resuscitation?

If not, this chapter is designed for you. Think of it as a first-aid map or as a detailed guide to the "top things to do BEFORE you treat the specific condition checklist" we discussed in Chapter 1. Here, you'll find step-by-step instructions used to take a pulse. You will also learn the basic procedures for treating a shock victim. By reading this chapter, you will be familiar with the five most necessary first aid skills. (The next five most important skills are covered in Chapter 4.)

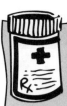

First Aids
The *pulse* is the movement of blood through the arteries. When the heart beats, the walls of the arteries swell with blood. Between beats, as the blood moves along, the walls shrink back to normal size. The rhythmic swelling and shrinking is what you feel when you take a person's pulse.

Take the pulse at the wrist.

Taking a Pulse

There are several different ways to take a pulse. If you can't feel a pulse at one location, you will need to try another area on the individual's body, as detailed in the following steps.

1. Place your second (index) and third (middle) finger on the inside of the injured person's wrist. Your fingers should be right below the wrist crease and near the thumb (see the following figure). Press down. If you find the pulse, go on to step 4; if you don't, proceed to the next step.

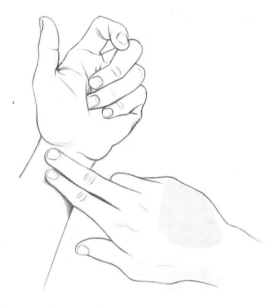

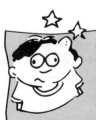

Ouch!
Never use your thumb to take a pulse. It has a pulse of its own, and what you feel while trying to locate a pulse may be your own beating heart and not the injured person's.

2. If you can't feel a pulse at the wrist, try the carotid artery at the neck as shown in the next figure. This is located below the ear, on the side of the neck directly below the jaw. You should feel the artery as you exert pressure on the neck. (This is the best place to take a pulse if you have to give mouth-to-mouth resuscitation.) If you find the pulse, go to step 4; if you don't, proceed with step 3.

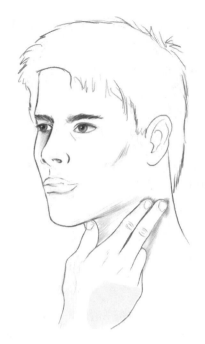

Take a pulse at the carotid artery.

3. If you still can't feel a pulse, try using the same two fingers on either side of the Adam's apple at the throat, the femoral pulse at the groin, or in between the muscles on the inner side of the upper arm.

4. As soon as you feel a pulse, count the pulse beats for fifteen seconds (you'll need a watch), exerting pressure with your two fingers the whole time.

5. Multiply the number you get by four. This gives you the individual's heartbeats per minute, or pulse rate.

A normal pulse ranges from 60 to 90 beats per minute. Babies can have pulse rates up to 120 beats per minute; young children's pulses range from 80 to 160.

A rapid pulse can be a sign of shock or severe strain on the heart such as an asthma attack or electrocution. If the beats are very faint or weak, an injured person might be in shock, his blood flow might be restricted, he might be in a hypothermic condition (from the cold), or he might be suffering from several other conditions. The main thing to be aware of when it comes to a faint heartbeat is to keep an ear out and keep an eye on the person's breathing. If the heartbeat is slow and is combined with ragged, almost nonexistent breathing, an emergency situation is definitely in

> **First Things First**
> If the pulse you find is very erratic, don't rely on math. Take a full 60 seconds to count the beats.

progress. You might have to perform CPR (if you are trained and certified) or mouth-to-mouth resuscitation until help arrives.

Practice taking a pulse on yourself or a family member so you'll be familiar with the process in case of an emergency.

Listening to the Heartbeat

Listening to an injured person's heartbeat is just as important as taking his or her pulse. Obviously, a heartbeat means the person is alive—even if the pulse is so weak that you can't feel it at any location. Here's how to listen to a heartbeat.

1. For men: Put your ear below the breastbone, slightly to the left of the left nipple.

   For women: Put your ear right below the left breast.

   For children: Put your ear slightly to the left of the left nipple.

2. Count the heartbeats you hear for one full minute.

A normal adult heart beats between 60 and 90 beats per minute. Children and babies can have ranges higher. When a heartbeat is too fast, it can mean the victim is suffering from agitation or panic, shock, or fever. Treat each of those conditions as needed.

Stopping Bleeding

Bleeding doesn't always signal an emergency situation. A minor cut doesn't have the same priority as an injury that creates profuse bleeding. No matter what the situation may be, there is one important rule to remember when it comes to treating wounds:

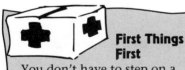

First Things First

You don't have to step on a rusty nail to get a tetanus (lockjaw) infection. Any wound is susceptible. The best preventative medecine is a tetanus injection every 10 years for everyone in the family. This is expecially important if you enjoy outdoor vacations or do extensive traveling abroad.

Always wash your hands before performing first aid to prevent infection. If soap and water aren't handy, make sure you have "wet naps" in your first aid kit.

Although you don't have to take extreme precautions when it comes to your immediate family, remember that with friends, colleagues, and strangers, it's always best to follow universal safety guidelines to prevent transmission of the HIV virus and other infections via blood. Always wear two pairs of latex gloves, a mask, goggles, and an apron, if possible.

As an extra precaution, make sure any open wounds or cuts on your skin are completely covered before performing first aid.

Where the bleeding is coming from is more important than the amount of blood you see. A minor cut can create profuse bleeding—as anyone who has cut him- or herself shaving knows.

When you check an injured person's vital signs, don't forget to check for signs of bleeding. After you've washed your hands, attend to the wound. Is it near a major artery or vein, such as in the inside of the wrist, along the neck, on the torso area, at the inner thigh, or on the back of the calf? Is it serious enough for stitches? Does the cut appear to be close to the surface? After you've determined where the cut is located, you can take appropriate steps to stop the bleeding, as described in the following paragraphs. And, as always, don't forget your universal safety measures!

Minor Scrapes

Treating minor cuts is relatively simple. If you have a child, you've most likely been doing it for years! You can tell a cut is minor if it's near the surface and is not close to any important veins or arteries.

Minor cuts can look a lot worse than they are. Here are some simple steps to follow when treating a minor cut:

1. Wash your hands to avoid introducing infection into the wound. Practice the universal safety measures as outlined in Chapter 2.

2. Wash the wound with an antibacterial antiseptic and a clean sterile cloth. In an emergency where help or a first aid kit are nowhere in sight, a *clean* ripped T-shirt will do! Only use an article of clothing in absolute emergencies because they are not always clean and may induce infection.

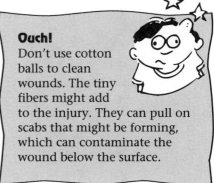

Ouch!
Don't use cotton balls to clean wounds. The tiny fibers might add to the injury. They can pull on scabs that might be forming, which can contaminate the wound below the surface.

3. Once you've applied a sterile cloth to cover the wound, apply direct pressure to the wound to slow the bleeding. Press firmly on the cut with your fingers and hand for several minutes without letting up. If the bleeding doesn't stop, you may have a deeper wound than you first thought. Get help as soon as possible. In the worst possible instance, you might have to apply a tourniquet.

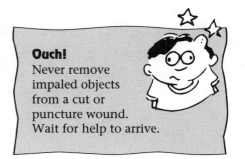

Ouch!
Never remove impaled objects from a cut or puncture wound. Wait for help to arrive.

4. After the wound stops bleeding, remove the pressure. Gently apply an antibiotic cream.

5. Cover the wound to avoid infection. Use adhesive bandages for small cuts and scrapes. Use non-stick gauze pads (taped down with adhesive tape) for large scrapes, surface area wounds, and wounds that are beginning to heal. Be careful when changing dressings because adhesives can pull on developing scabs.

Deep Wounds

Treating and cleaning deep wounds must be left to medical professionals only, but while waiting for help to arrive, you can still work to reduce bleeding. Apply pressure as described in the preceding section about minor scrapes. If the bleeding shows no sign of subsiding and continues to "gush" profusely, you might have to make a tourniquet. Tourniquets should be used only in life-or-death emergencies. Never use a tourniquet on the head, neck, or chest. Its unrelenting heavy pressure can stop the flow of oxygen to your heart, lungs, and brain—and cause permanent nerve and muscle damage. Tourniquets should only be used as a last resort for pulsing, spraying bleeding that cannot be controlled by direct pressure or elevating the limb. If you take a tourniquet off once you've put it on, bleeding could begin to flow twice as heavily as before. Always write down the time you applied the tourniquet and let the emergency squad know.

As a last resort, follow these steps to make a tourniquet.

1. Find a scarf, a piece of cloth, or a sheet that is at least two inches wide. Wrap the material just above the wound three times.

2. Tie the ends in a tight half-knot.

3. Place a stick, a piece of wood, a pen, a utensil, or anything that is between five and ten inches long directly on the knot.

4. Tie the ends of the cloth around the stick item to the tourniquet with a double knot.

5. Twist the stick until the bleeding stops or at least decreases to a minor "trickle." Do not twist any further, as you might do more damage.

6. Keep the stick secure with another tourniquet knot or with another piece of cloth.

Fickle, Thy Name Is Infection

Infection is a dangerous thing. Even after you've performed first aid measures exactly as described for cleaning wounds and stopping the bleeding from cuts, the victim is still not out of the woods. Infection can still set in, as much as hours or days after the injury.

In fact, infection is not just a problem with serious wounds. Minor wounds can also become infected, and can become so seriously compromised that it can lead to shock or coma!

Applying a dressing is not enough. You should be on the alert for signs of shock or infection so that when help arrives, the medical experts can begin treating for infection immediately. Signs of infection include:

The area around the wound feels hot.

The area around the wound is red.

The injured person feels pain at the wound site.

The wound site begins to swell.

Fever.

Chills.

To prevent severe infection and its fallout after the crisis is over, it's a good idea to change dressings on the wounds often and to check for signs of infection daily. If you notice any of the above symptoms of infection, treat them seriously! Call your doctor immediately and make an emergency appointment.

Performing Mouth-to-Mouth Resuscitation

If you've been certified and trained to do CPR, go to it at the first sign of breathing problems or an erratic heartbeat. But if you don't know CPR, do not attempt to try it during your first emergency. Instead, get help immediately. While you are waiting, try mouth-to-mouth resuscitation; it can help save a life. The following figure shows an example of how you perform mouth-to-mouth.

The following steps teach you how to do mouth-to-mouth.

1. First, ascertain whether the unconscious person is breathing at all. Bend down and place your ear near his or her mouth and nose and listen for signs of respiration. Look at his or her chest and see if you can see signs of exhalation. Hopefully, all is not lost and the person is breathing, even if it is faint.

2. Position the injured person on his back.

3. Put on latex gloves for universal safety measures. Open his or her mouth and use your fingers to remove any obstructions in the throat or airway, as shown in the top portion of the figure.

4. To avoid transmission of HIV or other deadly viruses via saliva, place your disposable airway bag over your mouth and over the injured person's mouth. (Obviously, if this is an intimate family member, you will not have to practice this universal safety feature.)

Performing mouth-to-mouth resuscitation.

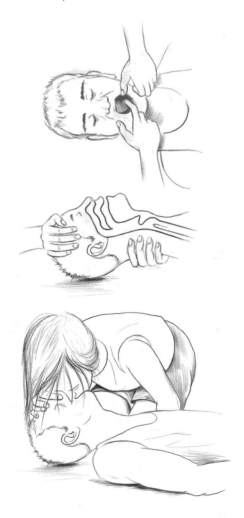

5. Put one hand under the injured person's neck, and place the other hand on his forehead. Tilt the head back as far as you can to keep the airway clear. The injured person's mouth should be open. (See the middle portion of the figure.)

6. Pinch the nostrils to close them.

7. Take a deep breath.

8. Cover the injured person's mouth completely with your own. (See the bottom portion of the figure.)

9. Exhale hard into the injured person's mouth. Repeat four times.

10. If you are working on an adult, stop for five seconds, and then repeat steps 6–9 giving only one breath.

   If you are working on a child or infant, stop for three seconds, and then repeat steps 6–9 giving only one breath.

11. Repeat this process until the victim begins breathing, until you feel a pulse, or until help arrives. During the time you're not breathing into the person's mouth, continue to call for help.

12. Remember the ABCs you learned in Chapter 1. Take a brief pause in-between your resuscitations to check the victim's Airways, Breathing, and Circulation.

Treating for Shock

When an individual goes into shock, the body's chemistry goes out of whack. Balance must be restored—quickly. There are different degrees of shock, but expect some obvious symptoms whenever an accident occurs. Signs of shock include:

Weakness	Nausea
Clammy, pale, cold skin	Chills
Erratic breathing	Faintness or unconsciousness
Weak and/or fast pulse	

If a victim goes into shock, don't panic. Perform the ABCs of first aid: clear Airways, check Breathing, and maintain Circulation. Cover the injured person with a blanket to keep her warm. Then lay her down, keep her quiet, and elevate the feet to maximize blood flow to the brain.

Above all, get help as quickly as you can.

The Least You Need to Know

➤ To find a pulse, use two fingers and press lightly at the wrist or carotid artery below the jawbone. Then count the pulses for 15 seconds. Multiply by four to get the pulse rate.

➤ A heartbeat means that circulation is "alive and well" and oxygen-rich blood is being pumped to all the cells. If you don't feel the heartbeat when you take a pulse, begin CPR (if you've had training to do so).

➤ You stop bleeding in most wounds by applying direct pressure over the dressing. If the bleeding does not stop and, in fact, continues to gush, make a tourniquet. (Wrap a piece of cloth or belt tightly about an inch above the wound.) Do not remove the tourniquet until help arrives!

➤ Whether a person experiences a deep wound or a minor cut, infection is always a danger. Cleanse with an antibacterial cream and cover with a sterile bandage. Change the dressing regularly, and inspect for signs of infection daily.

➤ Before performing mouth-to-mouth resuscitation, ascertain whether the person is inhaling and exhaling.

➤ When performing mouth-to-mouth resuscitation, use universal safety measures, including latex gloves and disposable airway bags to prevent the spread of disease.

➤ When a person goes into shock, his or her body chemistry becomes imbalanced. Signs include clammy skin, nausea, chills, and faintness. Reverse the imbalance by practicing your ABCs: Keep Airways clear. Help Breathing with mouth-to-mouth resuscitation. Maintain Circulation by loosely covering the person with a blanket.

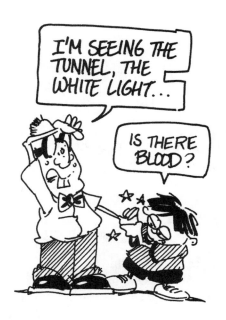

Chapter 4

Vital Emergencies: The Next Top Five "How Tos"

> **In This Chapter**
>
> ➤ Bandages for wounds from head to toe
>
> ➤ Immobilizing a patient with back and head injuries
>
> ➤ Slings for arms, fingers, and legs
>
> ➤ Keeping an injured person from panicking
>
> ➤ Treating bladder or bowel accidents

In many ways, you do have the tools you need to help an injured person until trained help comes along. Thanks to the principles you learned in the previous chapter, and you know how to take a pulse, and you know how to stanch bleeding. You can also determine whether a *real* emergency is at hand—or if the person can be helped with a clean dressing and a calm voice.

It's now time to learn the last five vital first aid "how tos" that you'll need to handle in the case of an emergency. By the time you finish this chapter, you'll be armed and ready for any contingency that may occur. (See Part 2 for descriptions of emergency situations and accidents that range from A to Z—and how to handle each one.)

Bandaging Wounds

Bandages have three purposes: to keep wounds clear of infection, to contain bleeding, and to provide additional protection and support. Sterile gauze is preferable, but in an emergency just about anything will make a good bandage: scarves, T-shirts, socks, sheets, stockings, even a belt.

Bandaging a deep wound requires more than simply sticking a Band-Aid over the cut and hoping for the best. Deep wounds require bandages that are administered after a wound is cleaned and treated at the hospital.

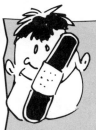

Before You Put the Band-Aid On

Never wrap a bandage too tightly. You want to keep bleeding in check and protect the wound, but you *don't* want to stop circulation or cause irritating chafing! If the wound is on an arm or leg, check circulation by making sure fingers or toes stay warm and pink. If they become cold or blue, it's a sign there's a circulation problem. Periodically check the patient's pulse just to make sure everything's okay.

Bandaging Head Wounds

If a wound affects the scalp, the bandage should be made by tying a kerchief on the head and knotting it in the back.

1. After putting on your protective gloves, stopping any bleeding, and cleaning the wound (see Chapter 3), fold a large bandanna-sized cloth into a triangle.

2. Place the bandage on the injured person's head, with the tip at the back.

3. Bring the two ends across the head, just above the ears and cross them in back.

4. Bring the two ends back to the center of the forehead. Tie ends together.

5. Tuck hem of bandage snugly under wrap.

If a wound only affects the forehead, put a square of sterile gauze pad over the wound. Then wrap a sterile gauze bandage around the head, "sweatband" style, as shown in the following figure. Circle the head at least three times to keep the dressing underneath in place. Cut and use adhesive tape to attach the ends, or tie them with a firm knot. You can also use a large piece of cloth, wrapping it several times around the head. Tie the ends in place above the eyes in the middle of the forehead.

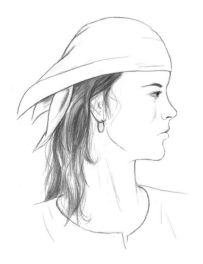
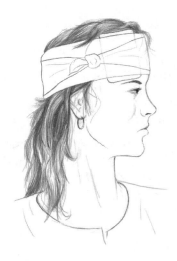

Bandages for large head wounds (left) and forehead wounds (right).

Ears and cheeks require a bandage that is more like an "old-fashioned toothache" style. These steps teach you how to apply such a bandage. The following figure illustrates the procedure.

1. Place the long, thick bandage under the chin.

2. Pull the ends up over the ears and cheeks, covering the treated wound.

3. Cross the ends on one side, just above the ear.

4. Wrap the two ends in the opposite direction, making a "cross" by encircling the forehead and back of the head.

5. Tie ends where the "cross" meets.

Ouch!
Do not use this bandage style if the injured person has a jaw problem or if he or she is vomiting. It can cause suffocation!

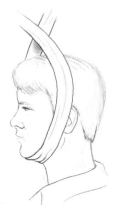
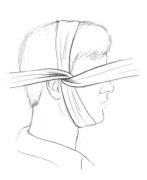
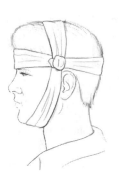

To bandage an ear or cheek wound, start by wrapping "toothache" style. Then cross the ends on one side of the head and tie on the other side.

Wrapping Knee and Leg Wounds

To make a bandage that won't come apart on the knee or leg, follow these steps:

1. Clean and dress the wound while wearing protective gloves.

2. Bend the knee unless it causes pain. Then place the middle of your wide, long cloth at the underside of the knee joint (and over any dressing).

3. Wrap the cloth, with opposite ends crossing, over the knee and the upper or lower leg (depending on the location of the wound). See the following figure for example.

4. Tie ends into a knot.

5. Secure the bandage with adhesive tape or safety pins.

Wrap the knee and upper leg.

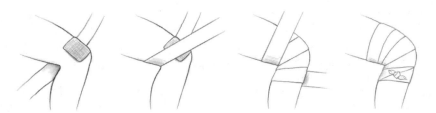

Follow these steps to apply a bandage to the leg using a spiral technique:

1. After you clean the wound and apply an antiseptic, place one end of a long, wide cloth on the outer side of the leg. Secure it with adhesive tape.

2. Twirl the bandage around the leg until you've covered the wound and dressing and the entire wound is protected.

3. Secure the loose end with tape or safety pin to keep in place.

Covering Arms and Elbows

Bandaging an arm or elbow is very much like bandaging a knee or a leg. Once you've cleaned and dressed the wound with an antiseptic cream, follow these steps:

1. Bend the elbow you're wrapping.

2. Place the center of the cloth in the crook of the arm.

3. Circle the two ends around the upper or lower arm (depending on the location of the wound). Then knot and tie it.

You can also use the "spiral" technique for an arm. To do so, anchor one end of the cloth to the outside of the arm with tape, and then wrap the other end around the arm's wound, over and over. Secure the other end with adhesive tape or a safety pin.

Bandages for Wrists and Ankles

Think of an ice skater performing a figure-eight. That same twisting technique is effective for bandaging wrists and ankles. Here's how you wrap a wrist (after cleaning the wound).

1. Tape one end of a long, clean cloth or gauze roll to the palm of the injured hand.

2. Roll the gauze or cloth two or three times around the palm of the hand.

3. Bring the gauze or cloth across the palm of the hand and then in-between the thumb and first finger.

4. Pull the gauze diagonally across the outside of the hand to the wrist (see the following figure).

5. Circle the wrist two or three times with the cloth.

6. Repeat steps 1–5 until the wound and dressing are covered. Then secure the bandage at the wrist with adhesive tape or a safety pin.

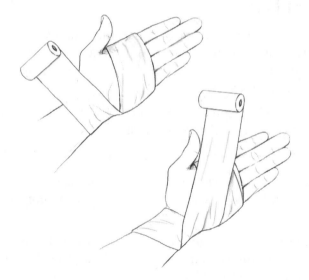

Wrap the bandage around the palm and then the wrist.

Follow these steps to use the same technique for wrapping an ankle:

1. Tape one end of a long, clean cloth or gauze roll to the instep of the injured person's foot.

2. Roll the gauze or cloth two or three times around the foot, moving from the instep to the back of foot, and from the back of foot to the instep.

3. Then bring the cloth up across the front of the foot and around the ankle (as shown in the next illustration).

4. Repeat this five to seven times.

5. Add one final circle around the ankle.

6. Secure at the ankle with adhesive tape or a safety pin.

Bandage the instep and then the ankle.

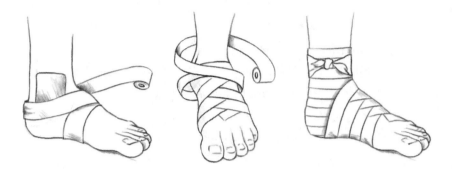

Bandaging the Back and Neck

When someone suffers an injury to the back or neck, it's more important to keep him or her immobile than anything else. But sometimes that's not possible. Maybe the victim is face down in water and cannot breathe. Maybe he is vomiting and needs to have his head tilted. Maybe this person is bleeding profusely.

As is true of grammar, there are always exceptions to the rules. In those situations when bandaging a back or neck wound is necessary, follow these steps:

1. Move the injured person as little as possible.

2. If cleaning and treating a wound is sufficient to stop the bleeding, simply put a loose cloth over the treatment. It will provide protection without adding possible trauma.

3. If an injured person feels a tingling in her limbs or cannot move, it's possible that she might have broken bones. In this case, immobilize the head, neck, and back area. (See the section about immobilization later in this chapter.)

4. If the injured person is having difficulty breathing, very gently lift his or her head slightly and place a pillow underneath. This will help clear air passageways.

5. Keep bandages simple. Use a "spiral" technique or cover the area and tape it down with some adhesive—just tight enough to stop bleeding.

6. Keep checking the injured person's pulse. If it starts feeling weak, loosen the bandages!

Wrapping Fingers and Toes

Bandaging wounded fingers or toes is just like bandaging any other part of the body but with smaller actions and smaller pieces of cloth. It also requires a bit more dexterity and it would be a good idea if you practice on a (willing) friend or family member *before* an emergency arises. After you clean the wound, follow these steps to wrap a finger or toe:

1. Using a long roll of narrow gauze or a strip of cloth, place one end at the base of the finger or toe.

2. Hold the strip down with your thumb as you roll up one side of the finger or toe and down the other side.

3. Hold the other side down with your third finger (or whatever fingers you feel comfortable using) as you roll the tape up and over with the other hand.

4. After wrapping several layers of tape up and down the finger or toe, move the gauze roll to the side and begin to circle the finger or toe.

5. Knot the gauze at the base of the finger or toe as shown here.

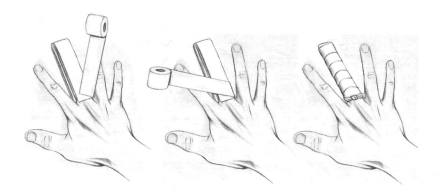

To bandage a finger or toe, first roll the gauze up and down, and then wrap the gauze around the digit. Finally, knot the bandage to complete the process.

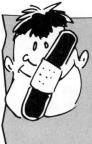

Before You Put the Band-Aid On

A splint immobilizes an injury to prevent further damage and to help promote healing. If a plastic or wooden brace is not readily available, the next best splint for a finger is the adjacent finger! Just be sure to place sufficient padding between the fingers before gently wrapping the fingers together.

A finger or toe bandage can also act as a splint in a pinch. Once you've bandaged the finger or toe (up and down and side to side), pull the gauze roll down to your wrist or up to your ankle. Wrap around the wrist or ankle, and then pull back up and around the finger (or down and around the toe). Repeat several times and tie at the wrist or ankle. The following drawing illustrates how to wrap the hand in this way.

You can adapt a finger or toe as a splint.

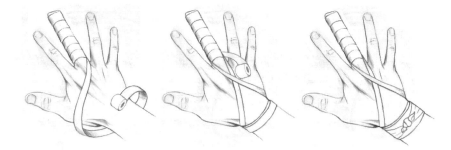

Immobilizing a Person with a Neck or Back Injury

The main reason you need to keep a person with a neck or back injury perfectly still is simple. Any movement, even the slightest bend or twist, can cause spinal cord damage. Neck and back fractures do not necessarily mean spinal cord injury, but undue movement can create a problem that may not have been there before. Spinal cord damage can result in permanent paralysis. The best position for an immobile person is flat on his or her back. But, if you find an injured person curled to the side or on the stomach, leave him or her in that position! Remember, there are only a few reasons to move a person, especially if he or she is unconscious.

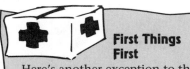

First Things First

Here's another exception to the "keeping an injured person immobile" rule. If someone is bleeding internally, it's important to roll him to the side to keep breathing passages open. Warning signs of internal bleeding include coughing up or vomiting blood, red or brown color in the urine, and red or black specks in the stool.

It's easy to tell someone to lie still, but what if he or she gets an itch or an unconscious twist? What if he or she contorts the body in pain? The best way to ensure immobility is to make a brace. Almost any bulky items will do. Rolled-up towels, newspapers, blankets, and purses are especially good. Use heavy items to keep the lighter, bulky objects in place. These can include luggage, books, plants in heavy clay pots, and cinder blocks.

If an accident occurs in the middle of nowhere and if the injured victim is unconscious with possible back or neck injuries, you can still move him or her with a modicum of damage. Gently roll the individual onto a board and pull him or her to safety. If there's no board, use a blanket. And, if there aren't any blankets handy, gently pull the injured person by the arms or ankles.

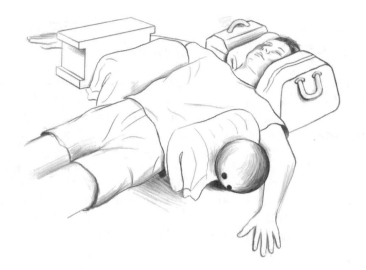

Use bulky and heavy items to immobilize an injured person.

How to Make a Sling or Splint

The "slings of outrageous fortune" might have created the emergency situation you find yourself in, but only a real, down-to-earth, and oh-so-practical sling will help you help someone with broken or bruised limbs. Here's an easy way to make an arm sling:

1. Fold a scarf or cloth into a triangle.

2. Put one end of the triangle at the shoulder of the uninjured arm. Let the triangle dangle down the chest.

3. Place the injured arm or bent elbow over the triangle dangling down the chest.

4. Pull the dangling portion of the triangle up to meet the end at the shoulder. The injured arm should be inside the triangle, elbow covered and fingers peeking out.

5. Tie the two ends together at the side of the neck—not at the back (you can damage the spine).

6. An ordinary safety pin will keep the sling in place. Using the safety pin, attach the point of the triangle at the elbow to the sling. (If you don't have a safety pin, twirl the point until the arm is snug, then make a knot.)

7. Make sure the hand is four to five inches higher than the elbow to keep the blood flow circulating and to decrease pain. Adjust the sling, if necessary.

See Chapter 21, "Muscle Cramps, Strains, Sprains, and Breaks," for more detailed information on slings, immobilization techniques, and combination bandages/slings to use on different body parts.

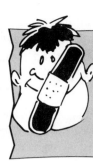

Before You Put the Band-Aid On

Letting the fingers peek out of a sling is not just to allow the injured person to wave hello. By having a clear view of the fingers, one can easily tell if circulation is being maintained. If the fingers turn pale or too red, adjust the sling or the bandage.

Like bandages, splints provide support to broken bones, fractures, sprains, and painful joints. When it comes to bones or joints, the most important first aid you can give is stabilization. This keeps those bruised and broken bones immobile so there is no further damage. Splints help the immobilization process. If you don't have actual boards in your first aid kit, use your imagination. Almost any hard, straight object will do. A rolled up newspaper or magazine, a baseball bat, a pillow, a folded blanket, an umbrella, or even a broom may be used to provide stabilization.

Ouch!
Don't tie the splint too tight. It can cut off circulation. While waiting for help, continue to check the splint. Make sure that post-accident swelling hasn't made the splint too tight. Also, periodically take a pulse. If it becomes faint, loosen the splint.

Regardless of what you use as a splint, it must be securely attached to keep the body part immobile. And, for secure attachments, don't go any further than the closet. Belts, ties, sleeves ripped from shirts, twisted-up T-shirts, stockings, and even underwear can be used as slings. They can easily reach around the arm or leg and be knotted, tied, or buckled securely. Table 4.1 contains suggestions for using basic everyday items to create splints for various body parts.

Use stiff items to create splints that immobilize joints.

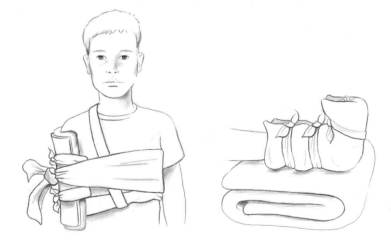

Table 4.1 Making Homemade Splints

Body Part	Splint Suggestion
Upper leg	Splint the two legs together.
Lower leg injury	Use a rolled up newspaper, a baseball bat, or a broom handle.
Ankles and feet	Rolled up newspaper or a magazine is best.
Back, Upper Torso, Head and Neck	Only hard earth will do. Immobilize the person by placing folded blankets and pillows up against him or her and securing them with belts, ties, or sleeves. Remember not to move a person if a back or head injury is suspected.
Arms	An umbrella, a stout stick, a cane, a baseball bat …any of these will work.
Hands	A small board, a notebook, a picture in a frame, magazines, or newspapers will give a hand support.
Fingers	Splint the problem finger with the adjacent finger.

How to Keep a Victim from Panicking

The best way to keep an injured person from becoming hysterical is to set an example. Remember the second principle of First Aid 101: Don't panic! If you stay calm, it will help the victim and other participating individuals stay calm. Even if you present a calm exterior (and the injured person can't hear your thumping scared-to-death heartbeat), the person who is hurt might be in terrible pain. He could be in shock, cold and trembling. He might be in and out of consciousness. But all is not lost. There are some techniques you can use to keep excess anxiety at bay.

Talk in a low, soothing voice. Be consistent and repetitive in your assurances. "Shh. You're not alone. I'm here. Help is on the way. Shh." Be reassuring but firm, kind but confident and assertive.

Get the person to talk. A good distraction will keep his or her mind off the accident. Talk about, say, your vacation, the weather, even a compliment on the great watch he or she is wearing. If it is someone you don't know, try to get a name and address and a family contact. Listen and nod your head. You can even ask about his or her feelings—if he is scared or if he is in pain, for example—but be objective. (Above all, don't yell!)

Use distraction, especially when you are treating wounds and applying bandages. Talk about the weather, yourself, or your family, or get the victim to talk.

If deep breathing works in normal day-to-day stress, there's no reason why it can't work in an emergency situation—as long as the injured person doesn't have breathing problems. Tell the victim to take a deep breath, count to four, and then exhale. Repeat this several times until the panic has subsided.

Trembling, crying, nausea, sweating, and mild gas pains are all typical reactions after an accident. Don't be too concerned about such things. However, if these symptoms don't pass, but instead get worse, act fast. Panic builds upon itself, and it is contagious. You don't need a group of panicked people trying to administer first aid!

How to Handle Bladder or Bowel Dysfunction

It might not be talked about in the latest episode of ER, but bowel and bladder accidents are common after an injury or traumatic experience. Fear, anxiety, and panic are emotional upsets and can manifest in physical ways. For many, the root of an injured person's dysfunction is not important. Whether it is a result of emotional distress or physical damage is irrelevant. The dysfunction should be treated as seriously as any other symptom. Calmly and with soothing words, clean up the mess using towels or cloths. Try to keep wounds clear of any bodily fluids or spills.

Above all, don't make a big deal about the situation. Embarrassment should be the least of a victim's problems during an emergency!

The Least You Need to Know

➤ Bandaging each body part has its own step-by-step instructions, but you can follow this general advice: Don't forget to wear your protective gloves. Always clean the wound, stop the bleeding, and dress a wound with antiseptic before bandaging it.

➤ If a head, neck or back neck injury is suspected, immobilize the injured person to prevent further harm. "Stuff" pillows, newspapers, and folded blankets up against the sides of the body and strap them in place with a belt or scarf.

➤ You don't need a plastic or wooden "official" splint to keep a broken arm or sprained leg in place. Be creative! Think baseball bats, umbrellas, canes, sticks, folded blankets, newspapers, or even a broom! Use the other leg or the next finger for a sturdy "hold," wrapping both the good appendage and the wounded one.

➤ Anxiety in an emergency is normal. Your job is to try to keep excess panic at bay. Use reassuring words, but be firm and confident. Even if you are nervous yourself, don't show it! Your nervousness will only heighten the victim's fear.

Chapter 5

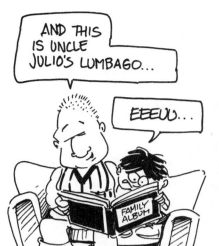

Your Family Medical History and Chart

By now, you are steeped in first aid lore. The ABCs of life support, Ace bandages, and Band-Aids dance above your head. You dream about splints, you can confidently handle vital emergencies, and you know how to stock the ideal medicine chest. But before we go on to specific emergency situations, I'd like to cover something that—although last in this part—is definitely not least in importance.

When it comes to first aid, the smallest factor can be of vital importance. Perhaps your child has an allergy to penicillin—and the emergency team that shows up is ready to inject. Perhaps a person's swollen throat is due to an allergic reaction to a bee sting—and not the asthma attack it looks like at first glance. Perhaps that swollen leg has nothing to do with a bad fall—but is an infection from a splinter that had never come out!

All of these factors can determine whether emergency first aid saves a life or causes more danger. And all of these factors also point to one thing: the necessity for a family medical chart that lists everything about everyone in your traveling troupe. If you keep a medical history handy (in a wallet, a pocketbook, or the glove compartment), you might be able to save a life if the need arises.

Using Your Family Medical History

How you react in an emergency situation greatly depends on your relationship to the person who needs help. When you help a stranger or someone you don't know intimately, following the safety guidelines for avoiding infection (to the best of your ability) is *de rigeur*. And you might even be able to treat the person without becoming emotional.

However, when the person who is hurt or injured is someone you love, everything changes. Though you may try to keep a clear head and not panic while you go through the first aid steps, your emotions play havoc and might actually interfere with your knowledge. Yet there is one major advantage to caring for someone you know well. You know the person who is hurt: you know who he is, what he is allergic to, what he is afraid of, and what the ramifications of the accident or injury can mean to him.

All of this information is part of a person's family medical history and should be documented in a family medical chart. A thorough medical chart is invaluable. Even though you may know your daughter's asthma symptoms or your son's allergy to bee stings like the back of your hand, having medical facts and history right in front of you will help you administer the proper first aid when your heart and head are at odds.

Everyone in the household should be aware that there is a chart and where it is. Consider putting a copy by every phone, in kitchen cabinets, in the bathroom by the medicine chest, in your car, and in your first aid emergency kit. You might also want one in the basement, by the fuse box, or near the ladder to the attic. In other words, keep a copy of the family medical chart accessible and handy.

Even better: everyone in the family should carry a list of his or her own allergies and current medications with him or her, just in case they're needed. This is especially important for children going to school, to summer camp, on an overnight trip, or to a sleep-over.

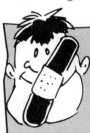

Before You Put the Band-Aid On

Medic alert bracelets and necklaces are vital for anyone in the family who:

➤ suffers from severe allergies or a chronic disease that requires special medication or treatment in emergencies

➤ has taken Prednisone (an anti-inflammatory medication) or Coumadin (for stroke patients) for three months or more

➤ has been diagnosed with diabetes, epilepsy, hemophilia and other bleeding disorders, or pituitary or adrenal deficiency

➤ has a pacemaker or a mechanical heart valve

Further, everyone in the family should be alerted to potential problem areas. Everyone from the youngest child to grandma should know about dad's bee sting allergies, mom's high blood pressure, older brother's diabetes. Be sure to let the baby-sitter, family friends, neighbors, and visiting relatives know what's what. And make sure your kids aren't afraid to tell emergency workers about a family history if they have to call 911. Come to think of it, make sure they know how to call 911, too!

Creating Your Family Medical Chart

To track family medical history, you should use a Family Medical Chart like the one in this chapter. If it's more practical for your family, create a separate chart for each family member, or use a small notebook or loose-leaf binder.

Before You Put the Band-Aid On

Always carry your emergency medications with you. A person with heart trouble has to have his or her nitroglycerin within reach. Asthmatics need inhalers, which is especially true for children who often "forget" or "run out of" their inhalers. Family members who are deathly allergic to bee stings need to be prepared (you can even be stung indoors). Frequently check to make sure that prescriptions are filled, that asthmatic inhalers are in good supply (and in stubborn children's lockers), and that bee sting kits are "fresh" and ready to use.

Whether you use a formal chart or you just keep medical records in a notebook, you should keep track of the following information:

➤ **Allergies.** For the same reason people wear medic alert bracelets and necklaces, writing down allergies on a family chart is vital for life-saving procedures. Emergency teams need to know about any contraindications with any medications and if a medication will make a patient worse instead of better.

➤ **Medications the person takes on a routine basis.** Contraindications are warnings you might find on the side of a medicine bottle or in the handout you receive from your pharmacist or physician; they mention possible health hazards involved if you take one particular medication with another one. An antacid, for example, is dangerous to someone who is taking tetracycline. Likewise, certain high blood pressure medications interact poorly with certain antibiotics. For these reasons, it's important to know what every family member is taking every day!

➤ **The family doctor's name, address, and phone number,** as well as that information for any specialist(s) the particular family member sees frequently.

➤ **A brief medical history that details previous or existing medical problems,** such as diabetes, heart disease, or epilepsy, and previously treated conditions, such as the insertion of a pacemaker.

➤ **Phone numbers for parents at work and for children at school.** If there is an emergency, a person must locate family members fast.

➤ **A neighbor's phone number and address.** If you have to rush one family member to the hospital, you might need the neighbor to pick up a package you've been waiting for or to watch the other kids when they get home from school.

➤ **An emergency phone number** (which might be the same as one of the others). Just in case that first number you list isn't working, or you're not working that particular day, or the person you mentioned to call in an emergency is in the Caribbean, it's good to have a second choice.

➤ **Date of last tetanus shot** (if none, that too should be noted).

In addition, it doesn't hurt to add a list of telephone numbers to the chart. Make copies of the chart, and each time you go out, you can add the number of where you'll be to that list. Then you'll have an up-to-date, complete list for the baby-sitter, too! This list should include numbers for:

Local poison control center (Poison needs its own fast "cure," which should be administered immediately—before help arrives. A poison control center will know much more than an ambulance driver about specific poisons, too.)

Local ambulance/hospital

Back-up ambulance/hospital (in case the first line is busy)

Police department

Fire department

Local pharmacy

Local taxi service (and a back-up service, just in case)

Nearby 24-hour drugstore (if not the same as the pharmacy). If you need to get an antibiotic or an antidote fast but it's three o'clock in the morning, it's nice to know you can still get help!

Gas and electricity companies' emergency numbers. If you smell gas or if sparks are flying from the lamp, you might need to call your local utility.

Family Medical Chart

Family Member	Allergies	Medical Problems	Medications	Date of Last Tetanus Shot	Phone Number at Work or School

Doctor	For Which Family Member(s)?	Address	Phone Number

Neighbor	Address		Phone Number

Telephone numbers:

Poison Control Center _____

Police _____

Fire Dept _____

Ambulance _____

Nearest Drug Store _____

24-hour Drug Store _____

Gas Company _____

Electric Company _____

Dentist _____

24-hour Taxi _____

Other _____

_____

47

The Least You Need to Know

➤ Make your own family medical emergency chart, and put it in every possible place you'll need to reach it fast: by every phone, by the medicine cabinet, inside a kitchen cabinet, by the garage door, and more.

➤ It's important to have your family's medical history down in writing for your baby-sitters, your neighbors, and your friends.

➤ A list of important phone numbers is vital. Some of them are self-explanatory: the police, the fire department, and an ambulance. But the local poison center is also important when seconds count.

➤ Back up numbers are also crucial. Find numbers for a back-up ambulance service, a taxi service, and emergency contacts such as a neighbor or friend.

Part 2
Simple, Safe, Step-by-Step First Aid

Consider this part a road map to first aid care. Alphabetized and categorized, the following chapters will help you in almost every circumstance. If your child gets stung by a bee, turn to the "Is" and the chapter on "Insect Bites—From Bee Stings to Ticks— and Other Skin Irritations." If your spouse is having trouble with his contacts, turn to the "Es" and the chapter on "Ear Aid, Eye Injuries, and Nose Damage."

On a much more serious note, if someone has a heart attack, you need to know what to do—and fast. Turn quickly to the "Hs" and the chapter on "Heart Attacks and Strokes." There you'll find step-by-step instructions telling you what you can do until professional help arrives. Combined with the general concepts you just read about in Part 1 of this book, the steps in this part just might help you save a life.

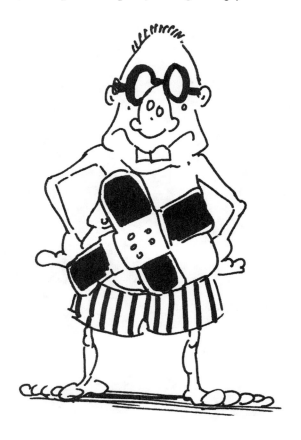

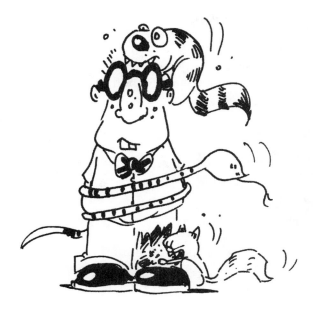

Chapter 6

Animal Bites, Scratches, and Snake Bites

> **In This Chapter**
>
> ➤ A rabid bite or a harmless nip?
>
> ➤ A snake!! Is it poisonous?
>
> ➤ "Mommy, Billy bit me." Treating human bites
>
> ➤ Treating and bandaging wounds until help arrives

We all love our animals, especially the pets that bring happiness to our families. But what about strange rabid dogs, slithering snakes, raccoons, and squirrels? This chapter will help you determine what to do when it comes to the bites and scratches created by "God's creatures."

Dog Bites and Cat Scratches

It might be true that household animals shouldn't "bite the hand that feeds them," but sometimes a pet dog or cat will lash out even at those they love—those who walk them, feed them, and hug them .

Most of these minor injuries can be treated with alcohol and anti-bacterial ointment. These injuries include the simple nips and scratches a dog might inadvertently cause while playing. Cats sometimes use their claws as a means to get your attention. Whatever the circumstance, these injuries are accidents, and if the animal in question has had its shots, there's no reason to be alarmed.

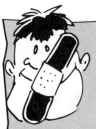

Before You Put the Band-Aid On

Some physicians have found cat scratch fever in patients complaining of fatigue, swollen glands, and flu-like symptoms. Sometimes a minor cat claw scratch can set off an allergic reaction or an infection, which causes the lymph glands to swell and creates flu-like problems. The symptoms of cat scratch fever usually do not last more than one week. If the symptoms last more than a week or worsen, contact a physician. If you have a fever, chills, or red streaks on your skin, you may need an oral antibiotic.

In order for an animal wound to qualify as a *bite*, it must break the skin. It doesn't matter if a person accidentally hits a dog's teeth or if a cat scratches the skin. If the epidermis (skin) is broken, bacteria from the animal's saliva can seep into the open sore, which may result in infection. Animal bites can potentially be serious. For example, if a stray dog attacks someone on the street, or if a rabid cat has scratched an individual, first aid needs to be administered immediately. Use these steps to treat more serious injuries caused by animals:

1. Stop any bleeding.

2. Try to capture the animal, or if it's someone's pet, get the name and address of the owner. Be careful not to be the pet's next victim. If it appears the animal is a stray, leave it alone. Do not attempt to capture it.

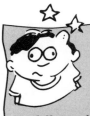

Ouch!
Do *not* use antibacterial lotion or cream on an animal bite. A bite is different from a cut or scrape; the bacteria in an animal's saliva can actually proliferate in certain creams!

3. Wash the wound for five full minutes. Running water is preferable, but if supplies are limited, you can soak the affected area in water that's frequently changed (of course, you'll be wearing protective gloves). This ensures that the saliva is completely washed from the wound.

4. Stop bleeding from minor cuts and scratches by adding direct pressure with a clean cloth. When possible, keep the injured area elevated above the heart. This will help control the bleeding.

5. Bandage the wound with sterile gauze and see a doctor the same day.

6. If the injured person has not had a tetanus shot within the past eight years, make sure a physician administers the shot immediately. *Any* bite can make a person vulnerable to tetanus (otherwise known as "lock-jaw").

The Danger Signs of Rabies

The only sure way to find out if a warm-blooded critter has rabies is to perform laboratory tests. However, there are certain signs that indicate the possibility of rabies. The following observations are often true of rabid animals:

➤ Wild animals come close to you instead of running away.

➤ The animal foams at the mouth, and its tongue hangs out.

➤ The animal can't seem to catch its breath; breathing is very labored.

➤ The wild animal suddenly lunges and snarls, ready to attack without provocation.

Rabies in its early stages is virtually undetectable, but there are some species that are more prone to rabies than others. If an untagged dog, bat, raccoon, skunk, fox, rat, or squirrel comes close to you, it is best to walk away slowly so as not to anger or frighten the animal.

Ouch!
Picture this scenario: A raccoon jumps out of the bushes and bites a friend you've been hiking with. Although your first thought is to kill the animal, you should really capture it instead. If you must kill the animal to defend yourself, try not to injure its head. Testing for rabies is conducted by examining the brain of potentially rabid creatures; that can be done even if the animal is dead.

Avoiding Injury to Yourself

There's an old saying that "If you're not good to yourself, you can't be good to anyone else." If you yourself get hurt by the same angry dog or nasty squirrel, you won't be much help to your companion. Here are some bits of advice that might help you avoid this predicament:

➤ Blow a whistle or yell loudly, and the animal should flee.

➤ If the person is not too badly bitten, carry or drag him or her to a safe place.

➤ This one's tough: Wait it out. As long as the animal is not continuing to attack, it's best to wait until he gets bored and leaves the scene completely.

53

➤ If you have no other recourse, if you are an expert marksman, and if you have a weapon available, kill the animal. But make sure the brain is not damaged so it can be examined for rabies.

Bites from Raccoons, Squirrels, Moles, Mice, Rats, and Other Small Critters

If one of these warm-blooded mammals attack, you should follow the same steps as for treating bites and scratches from dogs and cats. These animals tend to stay away from humans. If one does attack unprovoked, chances are it has rabies, so rabies treatments may be necessary. The good news? Treatment is much faster and less painful today than in the past. It doesn't require as many injections.

Children are especially vulnerable to bites from small animals. After all, raccoons and squirrels are adorable—and they even look like their favorite cartoon characters and stuffed animals. Unfortunately, these sweet-looking animals can, and will, bite to protect their hoard or their family. They will usually bite out of fear. If you are a parent, tell your children that these critters are wild and should be left alone.

Bears and Other Large, Wild Animals

Of course, your first instinct is to run. But sometimes the first instinct is not the best one. Some bears and other wild animals can run faster than you can, and some can even climb trees. When it comes to large animals, the best *first* first aid is prevention.

Don't go to campgrounds where bears have been sighted. Avoid exploring where wolves roam. If you see animal excrement in an area that's perfect for your picnic, let the animals have "first pick" and find another picture perfect spot for yourself! Other precautions you can take include wrapping food well to prevent the aroma from attracting unwelcome guests. If you can't store your food in a car, try packing food in zippered bags and hanging the bags in a tree. And, just in case there might be a surprise during the night, make sure you're in a ranger-approved, supervised campsite.

If the horrible happens and a bear attacks, make sure you follow the suggestions given earlier in the section "Avoiding Injury to Yourself." When the animal leaves you, staunch any bleeding and seek help. It's also best not to take chances with large, wild animals. If someone is bitten, he or she should be tested for rabies and treated. (Unless, of course, authorities managed to capture or kill the animal, and tests showed no sign of rabies.)

Human Bites

Accidents can happen, especially among children. If someone you love is bitten by another person, make sure you wash the wound thoroughly to avoid any potential infection. Follow the same steps as you would for treating animal bites.

Although it would seem that a human bite would be considered less serious than an "alien animal attack," in reality, a human bite is more likely to become infected! If you are bitten by a human, make sure you contact your doctor or visit an emergency ward. You'll most likely need antibiotics to ward off possible infection.

And, for today's virulent world, here's some sobering advice: test for HIV and other communicable disease. It's a matter of practical advice and a solid safety measure.

The only time you will have more cause for alarm is if a stranger bites an individual. The stranger could have rabies or a communicable disease. The police should be summoned as quickly as possible and the felon apprehended. Biting is as much a dangerous crime as gunshot wounds, knife stabs, or punches.

Snake Bites

There are two types of snakes to be aware of: poisonous and nonpoisonous. But any kind of snake bite can cause a reaction, which might include the following:

Swelling or bruising	Shortness of breath
Pain at the bite site	Rapid pulse
Nausea	Weakness
Blurry vision	

Because snakes blend in so well with their environment, it's not always easy to spot one. Sometimes you may spot one, and it is too late. Snake bites do not have to be fatal, or even life-threatening. The followings sections provide some first aid tips.

You can tell a poisonous snake by its appearance and by its bite marks. Believe it or not, most snakes are NOT poisonous. If bitten, a person might experience some slight symptoms, including minor pain and nausea, but that's about it. However, as benign as a snake can be, its bite is still worse than its "rattle." ALL snake bites should be taken seriously. A person bitten should be taken to a hospital as soon as possible.

Bites from Nonpoisonous Snakes

The typical "garden-variety" snakes have no fangs or rattles. They can be any color, but are usually black, brown, and other earthy hues. Some have beautiful stripes or geometric patterns on their backs. If you get a chance to look closely at a harmless snake, you'll also notice they have round eyes and that their skin is a clear, unpatterned color from the eye to the nostril (or *pit*). Their teeth marks will leave an elongated arch shape but no fang marks. The following illustration shows a nonpoisonous snake and its bite mark.

Nonpoisonous snakes have round pupils and no fangs, pits, or rattles. The teeth marks are generally arch-shaped.

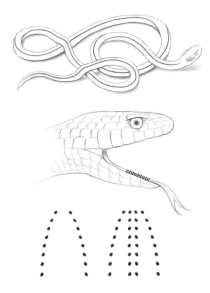

For proper first aid of bites from nonpoisonous snakes, follow these steps:

1. Call for help. Notify the local poison control center, and try to identify the snake. If you describe the snake to these experts, they can tell you if it is poisonous.

2. Make sure the injured person is lying down.

3. Soothe the injured person, keeping him or her as calm and as still as you possibly can.

4. If possible, keep the area that is bitten at a level lower than the heart. (Although this sounds dramatically poetic, it's vital medical fact.) If the bite is on the arm, keep it down. If the bite is on the neck, keep the victim in a prone position. And if the bite is on the leg, make sure it isn't elevated. In other words, no sitting up and adhering to gravity's pull. Why? Keeping the bitten area lower than the heart slows the circulation of the venom.

5. Tie a strip of cloth (scarf, watchband, or belt) about four inches above the bite site. It should be tight enough so that blood (and venom) will ooze out of

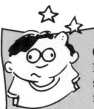

Ouch!
Never give alcohol, sedatives, or any form of aspirin to a person who is suffering from a snake bite. These medications can be harmful when combined with venom. Also, never use cold water, ice, ice packs, sprays, or cold compresses on the bite site. Cold can "disguise" swelling—which can be a life-threatening symptom that needs immediate first aid care.

the bite, but not so snug that you cannot feel a pulse. A good rule of thumb: If you can fit one finger under the strip, it's just right.

6. Wash the bite thoroughly with lukewarm water and soap.

7. Blot dry but do *not* cover.

8. While you're waiting for help to arrive, periodically check the person's pulse and the strip of cloth near the bite. Adjust as necessary, but do not remove.

9. If the area begins to swell, add another strip of cloth, four inches higher than the first and remove the first strip.

Identifying Deadly Pit Vipers

Did you know that an increasing number of reported snake bites in the United States come from imported "pets?" It's true. Some of these foreign animals, such as Puff adders and King Cobras, are more toxic than their North American counterparts. In fact, in the state of Indiana alone, more than one King Cobra bite has recently been reported! There are three kinds of poisonous pit viper snakes indigenous to North America. In general, you can quickly identify pit vipers by their triangular heads and tiny holes, or "pits." More specifically, you can distinguish among these deadly snakes by their descriptions, symptoms, and bite mark appearance.

The **rattlesnake** ranges from one to eight feet in length. Its distinguishing element is the rattle on its tail, which literally "rattles" before it attacks. It has large fangs, slit-like eyes, and tiny holes between its nostrils and its eyes. You can see the rattlesnake's rattle in this drawing.

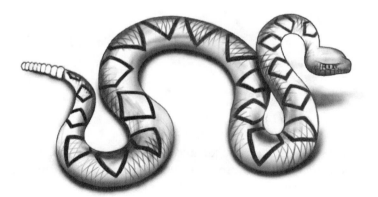

Rattlesnakes have a distinctive rattle.

Different types of rattlesnakes are found across America and Mexico. They are especially prevalent on the east coast, from Canada to Argentina. Rattlesnakes can be found as far north as New Hampshire and are somewhat common in the vicinity of Kansas and Oklahoma.

Rattlesnake venom attacks the circulatory system. The snake's long fangs can't help but enter the skin at an angle, which makes drawing out the venom a much easier task. (You'll learn about treating poisonous snake bites later in the chapter.) Rattlesnake bite symptoms include:

Severe pain and blood blisters at the site of the bite

Rapid swelling in the area of the bite

Numbness or paralysis in body parts close to the bite

Rapid pulse or a very faint pulse

Difficulty breathing

Shock or convulsions

Slurred speech

Pinpoint pupils or blurry vision

Unconsciousness

Conspicuous bite marks: two fang imprints plus teeth marks

Ouch!
They might not be as fast as a speeding bullet, but snakes are fast and can bite two extremities (an arm and a leg or two arms or two legs) in a flash! Always check the entire body for a second bite.

The following illustration shows the bite mark of a pit viper. Sometimes only one fang of a pit viper breaks the skin, leaving an odd bite mark.

A typical bite mark impression for a pit viper (rattlesnake, copperhead, or water moccasin).

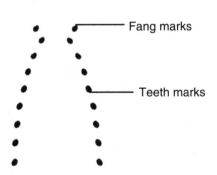

Fang marks

Teeth marks

Copperheads are also known as adders, pilot snakes, and highland moccasins. They have a bold geometric pattern along their body, and they are "chunky," reaching only about four feet. Like the rattlesnake, they have slits for eyes, two fangs alongside their teeth, and a pit on each side of their heads.

Look for (or, rather, *don't* look for) copperheads from Massachusetts to Illinois. You can also find them in the southern states, including West Texas. For some reason, they leave Florida alone, preferring to "vacation" elsewhere.

Also like the rattlesnake, a copperhead's venom attacks the circulatory system, and their long fangs enter the skin at an angle, which makes drawing the venom out a much easier task. Unfortunately, copperheads strike fast, and they don't give the "rattle" warning before they bite as rattlesnakes do. Copperhead bite symptoms are the same as those of rattlesnakes. See the list in the section on rattlesnakes. The next illustration shows a copperhead.

The **water moccasin**, also known as the cottonmouth, is a vicious pit viper. Like the copperhead, it is "chunky" and reaches a length of only four feet. As with all pit vipers, it has slit-like eyes, two fangs, and a pit on either side of its head. It is found in freshwater swamps, shallow lakes, sluggish streams, and river banks. Water moccasins like to live in the Southeastern sections of the United States. Because they can glide through water, water moccasins can quickly sneak up on an unsuspecting person and easily strike a toe or finger. Bite symptoms and bite mark impressions for water moccasins are similar to those of the copperhead and the rattlesnake. Their venom also attacks the circulatory system and their long fangs enter the skin at an angle. Again, this makes drawing the venom a much easier task.

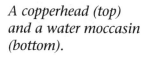

First Aids
Many of these dangerous species are also called *pit vipers* because of the tiny hole, or pit, they have on either side of their narrow heads. Rattlesnakes, copperheads, and water moccasins are pit vipers.

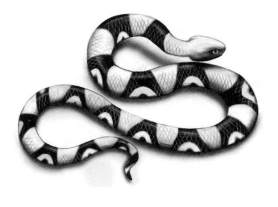

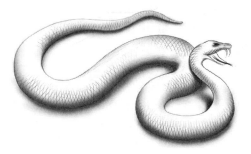

A copperhead (top) and a water moccasin (bottom).

Another Deadly Type: Coral Snakes

The fourth kind of poisonous snake to be aware of is the coral snake. Coral snakes are the most deadly poisonous snakes in America. Relatives of the hypnotic Cobra in India, coral snakes bite without leaving a fang mark. They have very short fangs and "chew" with their teeth (they are not pit vipers). Unfortunately, this enables the venom to spread faster and wider.

Coral snakes are beautiful to behold. As you can see in this illustration, their skin consists of bold black and yellow rings. They have black noses and round eyes, and they are short—only about three feet in length. Although they prefer tropical climates, you could find corals in the Gulf states, Texas, New Mexico, and Arizona.

The colorful coral snake.

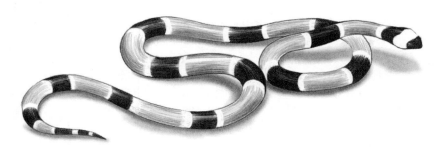

Coral snake venom affects the nervous system. Thus, the symptoms from their bites are different than those of a pit viper bite. Symptoms of a coral snake bite include:

Minor pain and swelling at bite site	Inability to speak
Droopy eyelids and blurred vision	Difficulty breathing
Drooling	Paralysis
Sleepiness	Shock
Voluminous sweating and chills	

First Aid for Poisonous Snake Bites, Step-by-Step

If medical help is nearby, follow the first aid steps for nontoxic snakes and get the person to a hospital as quickly as possible. But, if medical help is more than an hour away, you will have to perform some lifesaving techniques of your own. If you live in or are vacationing in an area that's known to have snakes, be sure to carry a snake bite kit in your emergency first aid kit.

In the past, making incisions and extracting venom was the acceptable mode of emergency care. But newer guidelines from poison control centers do not recommend that you make an incision or extract venom. Never make an incision for a coral snake bite. Because their bite is more of a chew, and fang marks are absent, you can actually spread the venom throughout the body. For a coral snake bite, use the first aid procedures for nonpoisonous snakes.

The only times you should perform that extreme type of care is when help is more than one hour away. Even then, you should do it only if you have an unopened, unused snake bite kit with a suction device. If you find yourself in that situation, follow these life-saving measures to make incisions and extract venom:

1. Sterilize a knife or razor blade by skimming it over a lighted match several times.

2. Carefully make a 1/2" vertical cut directly above each fang mark. Keep the incision shallow.

3. The suction cup portion of your snake bite kit looks like a small rubber ball. Squeeze it several times to get the air out. Then squeeze and hold it and place it over the bitten area; it should form an airtight suction. Follow the directions in your kit to extract the venom. (You'll be literally "pumping" the venom out.)

4. Provide suction for 30 minutes.

5. Wash the bite area thoroughly with soap and lukewarm water. Blot dry.

6. Keep checking the pulse of the injured person. If he goes into shock or stops breathing, follow the steps in Chapter 1 for giving mouth-to-mouth resuscitation and treating shock.

Ouch!
If you don't have a suction cup, you can suck the venom out by using your mouth. This is called incision, and it is controversial. Attempt it only if you do not have any other options. And never perform it if you have open wounds or cuts in your mouth. HIV can be a serious threat in this situation. Therefore, you should *always* carry a snake bite kit with you to avoid unnecessary risk to yourself and your peers!

The Least You Need to Know

➤ Always take the injured person to a hospital if a bite has broken the skin—especially if it's a human bite.

➤ Thoroughly wash bites with soap and warm water for five minutes.

➤ Remember the danger signs of rabid animals and stay away from any animal that you are unsure of!

➤ Know which snakes are poisonous and which are not. If you are familiar with snakes, you can save a lot of anxiety for the injured person.

➤ Never apply ointments, antibacterial creams, ice, or cold compresses on snake bites.

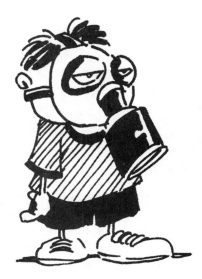

Chapter 7

Asthma Attacks and Other Breathing Problems

In This Chapter

➤ Handling breathing problems when seconds count

➤ Helping an asthma victim stay calm and comfortable

➤ Treating hyperventilation

➤ Dealing with an allergy attack

It's no laughing matter when you cannot laugh or speak or catch your breath. Breathing problems are particularly scary because they can be their own worst enemy: difficulty breathing creates anxiety, which makes the breathing problem worse!

If someone around you is having problems breathing, it's important that *you* stay calm. Practice the principles of first aid care you learned in Chapter 1: don't panic, call for help, check the pulse, and place the injured person in a position that's best for him or her to breathe and to keep airways clear. (Most likely, the best position to ease breathing is either sitting up or semi-reclining.)

Breathing problems range from hyperventilation to asthma to allergy attacks, each of which has its own first aid treatment. Whether the emergency occurs on the beach, in the house, or on the road, these conditions can appear worse than they seem—or they can be as dangerous as they appear to be! The best bet is to read through this chapter before a problem arises. You'll have a better feel for what to do when a breathing crisis occurs.

This chapter teaches you the ins and outs of the first aid care you need to give when asthma or another breathing difficulty occurs. If a person stops breathing entirely, see Chapter 3 for specific instructions on giving mouth-to-mouth resuscitation. Choking, which is a different condition from the labored breathing we describe here, is discussed in Chapter 9.

Helping the Asthma Sufferer to Breathe

When someone suddenly can't catch his or her breath, it's hard to stay cool. But that's exactly when calm, sound logic can mean the difference between life and death. Asthma is a common ailment; millions of Americans suffer its breathless slings. In many cases, someone having an asthma attack will know what to do. He or she may have an inhaler handy, which can aid breathing until help arrives.

But what if it's a child who suddenly can't catch her breath? Or a colleague or a stranger who doesn't have an inhaler at hand?

The first step is to recognize an asthma attack for what it is: it's not simply a case of hyperventilation. An asthma attack sounds terrible; a person is literally fighting to catch his or her breath. He might lean over, move around, or act quite agitated, or he might sit in a chair with his head back using all his body's energy to breathe. There might be a cough, a rasping of breath, or a rattle. Breathing itself will use almost the whole upper torso, the neck, the shoulders, and, of course, the mouth.

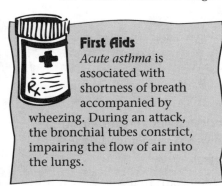

First Aids

Acute asthma is associated with shortness of breath accompanied by wheezing. During an attack, the bronchial tubes constrict, impairing the flow of air into the lungs.

If any of these signs occur, try to get help as fast as you can. If the person has an inhaler, use it! Although you cannot be sure an asthma attack is in progress, the longer you wait for help, the more serious the attack will become. Remember, asthma can kill if it is not treated early enough. Later on, even an inhaler won't help.

The main goal before help comes is to get a person to breathe as normally as possible. This is done through position, relaxation, and comfort.

Position: Have the victim sit up or lean back in a semi-reclining position, whichever is the most comfortable. Do *not* let the person lie flat; it can make breathing even more difficult. Use an inhaler if the person has one, or if you have one available.

Comfort: Loosen any clothing around the neck and chest.

Relaxation: Say soothing words and use calm motions to keep anxiety at bay.

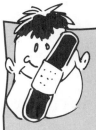

Before You Put the Band-Aid On

What appears to be an asthma attack could be congestive heart failure, one of the most serious causes of shortness of breath. This condition is exactly what it sounds like: the heart becomes congested with fluid as a result of something such as a heart attack or bronchitis or pneumonia that goes unchecked. If you're trying to decide whether a person is having congestive heart failure or a possible heart attack (see Chapter 17) and you need to perform heart injury first aid procedures, consider these things:

➤ **Age** The older the person, the more at-risk she is.

➤ **Medical history** If the individual can answer you, ask questions concerning medical history. Also look to see if he or she is wearing a Medic Alert bracelet.

➤ **Pain** Accompanying pain in the chest, arms, shoulder, or stomach can point toward a heart attack or possible congestive heart failure.

➤ **Sweat** Profuse sweating and clammy skin—even in freezing weather—go hand-in-hand with a heart attack or congestive heart failure.

And, whatever the medical facts, call for help. The cliché, "'tis better to be safe than sorry," is no more apt than when it comes to the heart.

Helping During Hyperventilation

Although its root might be anxiety, the sensations that accompany hyperventilation are very real. The sufferer may experience the sense of not catching one's breath, the feeling of overwhelming terror that something is wrong, and the feeling that there is a loss of control. Hyperventilation can mimic an asthma attack or a heart condition. It occurs during an acute anxiety attack. Symptoms can include:

Numbness in the hands, feet, and mouth

A tingling sensation in the fingers or toes

Overwhelming feelings of panic

Chest pain

Light-headedness

Inability to catch one's breath

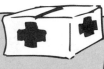

First Things First
Because it is difficult to distinguish between hyperventilation and asthma, find out if the party having difficulty has any history of anxiety disorder or asthma. If you can't get an answer, it's better to be safe than sorry. Perform first aid for asthma, making sure the injured person is comfortable and his or her clothes are loosened, before trying hyperventilation techniques.

Although these symptoms are very real, they are not the source of the problem. Overbreathing is the cause: A person literally breathes in too much oxygen.

To stop hyperventilation in its tracks, simply use a paper bag as described here:

1. Have the hyperventilating person breathe slowly into a paper bag that's held closely around his or her mouth and nose.

For hyperventilation, have the victim breathe into a paper bag for several minutes.

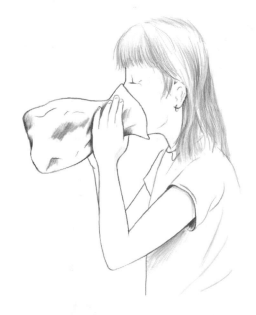

2. The person should breathe like this for five to seven minutes.

3. Talk to the individual the entire time. Try to distract him or her and make the person feel comfortable and safe.

4. If symptoms fail to improve or the person loses consciousness, take him or her to the emergency room.

First Things First

If you don't have a paper bag, plain old hands will do. Simply have the person cup his or her hands over the mouth and nose and breathe in and out for at least five minutes.

That's all it should take. When the person breathes back in the carbon dioxide that she just exhaled, the correct chemical balance in the blood is restored and the physical symptoms cease.

When a person hyperventilates, emergency medical assistance is usually not necessary if the procedures above are followed. But call a physician just in case; what looks like hyperventilation could be the onset of asthma or a severe allergic reaction that requires medication for relief.

Breathing Difficulties Resulting from Allergic Reactions

Parents often refer to this condition as croup. Health professionals call it allergies. These allergies affect the bronchial and respiratory systems. Rather than hives or itchy, red skin, allergies that affect breathing literally cause the throat to swell, making it difficult to inhale.

Symptoms of this type of breathing problem include wheezing, hoarseness, and a harsh cough. To give first aid for it, follow these steps:

1. Call for medical assistance.

2. If a shower is nearby, create a "steam room" by turning the hot water on high with the shower curtain closed. If the person is an adult, hold him or her upright so that the steam is focused on the face.

   If the affected person is a child, lift her on your shoulders and have her breathe in the steamed air. (Be careful not to let any of the hot water splash on either one of you!)

First Aids
Croup is, in actuality, a "reactive airway syndrome." A virus (or other infection) causes the airway to become overly sensitive and hyperactive to stimuli. This results in spasms in the airway and wheezing. Once the inflammation dies down (which can take several weeks), the airways become more normal. Antihistamines used to treat hay fever and allergies are not always effective in croup because the actual airways are in trouble as opposed to the entire bronchial system.

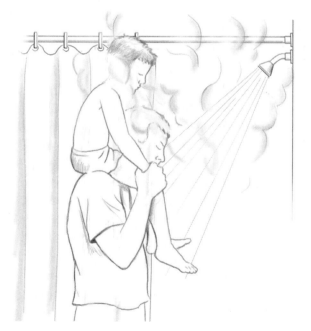

Use a "steam room" shower to help a child or adult having breathing difficulties caused by allergies (croup).

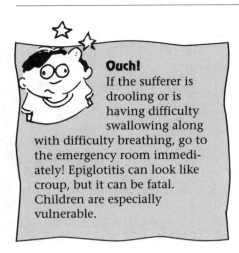

Ouch!
If the sufferer is drooling or is having difficulty swallowing along with difficulty breathing, go to the emergency room immediately! Epiglotitis can look like croup, but it can be fatal. Children are especially vulnerable.

3. Use your own judgment when it comes to steam. It can't hurt, but it might not be of any benefit either. If the steam helps restore breathing, keep the patient inside for up to 10 minutes, but never leave him or her unattended. Keep a vigil.

4. After the person having difficulty leaves the "steam room," have him or her lie down, head slightly uplifted. Towel the person dry and cover him or her with a warm blanket.

5. If the breathing problems begin anew, put him or her back in the steam. Continue the process until help arrives. (Unless it's a blizzard or a twister outside, this shouldn't take more than 20 minutes to a half hour!)

Sometimes the previous steps are all you need to clear breathing passageways. If the victim is starting to breathe easier, and you are at home and have access to a vaporizer, place it close to the person's bed. A good night's sleep might be all that's necessary.

Dealing with Dangerous Allergies

Sometimes allergic reactions can be more serious than asthma attacks, and seconds really count. A bee sting, an allergy to seafood or some other food (such as peanuts), or an allergy to certain weeds or flowers may be dangerous. Any of these can create an anaphylactic reaction, in which the throat swells so much that a person eventually won't be able to breathe at all.

The only recourse is to make the victim as comfortable as possible, to follow the first aid instructions for asthma and allergies, and get emergency medical help as fast as you can. (Call for an ambulance and the nearest physician.)

An epinephrine medication must be administered to neutralize the allergic reaction. People who have such allergies are usually aware of their symptoms. They sometimes carry epinephrine injection kits prescribed by their doctors for such emergencies.

If a person stops breathing before help arrives, mouth-to-mouth resuscitation is always an appropriate treatment (but don't perform it unless you've had professional training). Remember that breathing has stopped because of inflammation, congested airways, or a "deluge" of immune-resistant chemicals. Therefore, medication that decreases the inflammation and the harmful chemicals is the only thing that will work. Try an inhaler if the emergency becomes acute.

Don't forget the importance of a Medic Alert bracelet. It can contain vital information that could ease allergic reactions and even save lives.

The Least You Need to Know

➤ Recognize the differences between hyperventilation, asthma attacks, and allergic reactions. Although they may look the same, they require different treatment. If you are not sure which one a person is suffering from, don't wait to find out. Take him or her to a hospital.

➤ Asthma can be relieved by the use of an inhaler. But always seek help if asthma is suspected. The longer you wait to treat an attack, the lower the chances are that an inhaler will work.

➤ Hyperventilation can be relieved by breathing into a paper bag.

➤ Croup and other breathing difficulties can often be relieved with steam.

➤ Allergies can be life-threatening when the throat swells up so much that a person simply cannot breathe. An anaphylactic first aid kit is a good investment for your first aid kit, especially if someone in your family suffers from allergies!

➤ Handle potential life-and-death emergencies, such as heart attacks or anaphylactic reactions to allergies, by getting help as fast as you can. If an emergency medical team can come quickly, that's great. Otherwise, get in the car and go to the emergency ward yourself!

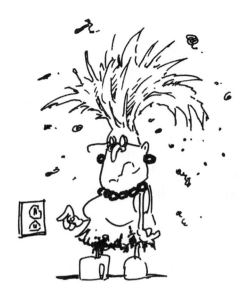

Chapter 8

Bumps, Bruises, Burns, and Electric Shock

In This Chapter

➤ Bumps and bruises: How they can be dangerous if not treated correctly

➤ Dealing with bleeding you can't see

➤ First-, second-, and third-degree burns: aid for all

➤ Treating for electric shock without hurting yourself

Bumps and bruises are the most common type of injury, and in most cases they require the least amount of first aid. Electric shocks are much more dangerous, and some of the worst shocks come from common household items and outlets. If you do not know the correct first aid procedures, you can actually make those bumps, bruises, burns, and electric shocks worse. You can even hurt yourself in the interim!

In this chapter, we'll go from the least serious to the most serious injuries, showing you first aid treatment step-by-step all the way.

Scrapes, Cuts, Bumps, and Bruises

Bumps and bruises are damage that occurs in the soft tissue under the skin. Under the following conditions, there is no need to call for medical assistance when a person suffers a cut, scrape, bump, or bruise:

➤ The injury is small (less than 1/2 inch around).

➤ There is no bleeding, or only slight bleeding. Make sure you follow the universal guidelines, such as wearing protective gloves, to prevent the spread of HIV or any other dangerous infections. (See Chapter 3 for first aid care for bleeding.)

➤ The victim is not in excessive pain.

➤ The victim does not feel numbness or tingling.

➤ The person is not suffering any paralysis.

➤ The victim does not seem to have any broken bones or dislocation at the joints. (If the victim is in a great amount of pain and the shoulder, leg, arm, or ankle appears to be lying or hanging at an awkward ankle, there is a good chance he or she has a broken bone or a dislocation.)

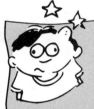

Ouch!
If the injury swells too much, the bump could signal a bone or joint injury. And, if the bruises keep coming too fast and furious, it could signal a more complicated medical condition.

Cut and Scrape First Aid

Here are simple first aid procedures for treating minor scrapes and cuts:

1. If the injured area has a skin scrape, wash it with mild soap and lukewarm water.

2. Apply Bacitracin or some other type of antibacterial cream or spray to prevent infection.

3. Cover the wound with a sterile gauze pad and tape or a simple Band-Aid.

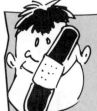

Before You Put the Band-Aid On

Bruises on the hands, fingers, feet, and toes can cause more problems than those that occur on knees, shins, or arms. Your hands and feet are a complicated network of motor functions, nerve endings, and flexibility. Any problems in these areas can cause a disability. For example, stubbing a toe might make walking difficult, or a damaged finger might keep you away from the computer. If you or someone around you experiences more than minor swelling or bruising after bumping into something or falling down, call your physician.

The Difference Between a Cut, a Bump, and a Bruise

A cut and a bruise, with or without swelling, are basically the same thing, except that one occurs at the body's surface, and the other occurs under the surface, in the soft tissue below the skin. In fact, the ugly black and blue marks you see when you bruise are really blood clots that form under the skin. The worse they look, the more they are clotting and healing.

But because bruises (and their potential partner, swelling) don't break through the skin, there is a difference in first aid treatment. Follow these steps for treating bruises.

1. Immediately apply an ice pack to the bruise to reduce swelling. (If an ice pack isn't available, use ice wrapped in a cloth or as cold a compress as you can make.)

2. If possible, elevate the bruised area so that it is higher than the heart. This keeps blood from "pooling" in the affected area (and thus creating more internal bleeding and swelling).

3. Keep the bruise elevated for approximately 15 minutes if the wound is minor. If the bruise is severe and it covers a large portion of the body, call for help. (See Chapter 4 for immobilizing techniques, if necessary; see Chapter 21 for information on treating sprains and breaks.) Keep a severe bruise elevated for at least an hour or until a trained emergency care team arrives.

4. If the bruise doesn't appear to be getting any better and more than 24 hours have passed, see your physician.

5. Seek prompt medical help if there is any swelling around the bruise, especially if it occurs at a joint. This can signal danger to nerves, muscles, and bones, all of which require a trained physician's attention.

> **First Aids**
> A *blister* is a built-up, fluid-filled irritation under the surface of the skin. A *blood blister* is a red blister that contains blood. A *fever blister* is another name for a cold sore or a herpes simplex at the lips. None of these are dangerous, but if they are accompanied by excessive pain or fever or if they grow larger, you should see your physician for proper drainage and possible medication.

The Warning Signs of Internal Bleeding

A slight amount of bleeding that creates a bruise under the skin is one thing, but hemorrhaging is quite another. Internal bleeding can be serious and can affect one's vital organs. The symptoms of internal bleeding are similar to those of shock:

➤ Pale, clammy skin

➤ Chills

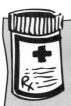

First Aids
Hemorrhaging is another word for uncontrollable bleeding. Because it is caused by breakage in blood vessel walls, it is usually internal, which means you can't always tell that a person is (literally) bleeding to death!

➤ Cold hands and feet

➤ Dilated pupils

➤ Rapid, weak pulse

➤ Major swelling at the injury site

➤ Major or immediate black and blue marks at the wound

Unfortunately, first aid procedures will not stop internal bleeding. The best thing to do is to call for help immediately. Then proceed with the first aid steps for shock (see Chapter 3).

First Aid for Burns

Burns are ugly, they hurt, and they are scary. But they can be treated with simple first aid steps. In fact, they are the one injury that *must* be treated before medical help arrives. The fact is that burns, unless treated right away, will get worse. They'll get deeper below the surface of the skin because the heat continues to do damage.

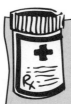

First Aids
When it comes to burns, *degree* has nothing to do with temperature. The terms first-, second-, and third-degree identify the severity of a burn. Of those, first-degree is the least harmful, and third-degree is the worst.

You might not think of your skin as an organ; after all, it hardly looks like a kidney or a heart. But the skin is a system of the body, and it's the largest organ of the body, too. It's the first shield against aliens, a natural-growing, one-person army of protection, germ warfare, and elimination. If something happens to the skin, the rest of your body is much more vulnerable to infection, shock, and disease. A burn, which affects that skin, is its worst nightmare come true. Unless you act fast, a burn can seep into the skin and invade your entire body.

The next few sections cover each degree of burn and specific first aid treatment for it.

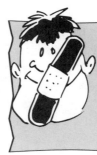

Before You Put the Band-Aid On

Because first aid treatment depends on a burn's severity, it's important to correctly identify the severity of the burn. Check the appearance at the *center* of the wound. That's usually where the burn is deepest, which is your indicator of what degree of treatment is required.

The Three Goals in Treating Burns—No Matter the Degree

There is a light (excuse the pun) at the end of the tunnel when it comes to burns. The fact is that burns can be treated successfully if first aid is administered quickly. By reading this section of the book, you are already ahead of the first aid burn game. You will know how to act fast in case of emergency. You will know how to treat a burn, regardless of the degree or cause, while you wait for help to arrive.

1. Prevent shock.

2. Ease pain.

3. Reduce the risk of infection.

The "Thou Shalt Not" Commandments for Burn Treatment

The first aid measures you *don't* take can be as important as those you do take, especially when it comes to burns. For example, earlier in this chapter, you learned that treating bruises is different than treating cuts, despite the fact that you can follow basic, general outlines for both. In short, there are always exceptions to every rule. And, when it comes to burns, these exceptions can save a life! Here's the "short list" on what not to do:

➤ Do not pierce or open blisters. It leaves the burned person "wide open" for infection.

➤ Do not peel off burned dead skin. It not only leaves the new skin underneath too vulnerable to infection, but it can cause scarring.

➤ Do not attempt to peel away any clothing stuck to the burn. Pulling away the cloth can also peel away any healing skin. And, as anyone who's ever had a bandage pulled off knows, it can hurt too!

➤ Do not use butter, antiseptic creams, or any other "folk remedies" on burns. They can actually *cause* the infection you're trying to avoid! None of these remedies, especially butter, will do anything beneficial for major burns.

Ouch!
It's one thing to fantasize yourself a hero, but unless you are a trained firefighter or medical professional, you should leave the saving to those who know how. Backdrafts, fallen rafters, smoke inhalation, and related hazards can affect you too—and instead of being a hero, you may become a victim. The best heroic deed is to get help fast.

In the First Degree

Accidentally touching a hot burner, getting too much tropical sun, and holding a scalding hot pot are all ways you can get first-degree burns. First-degree burns are the most benign and most common burns of all. However, because first-degree burns irritate nerve endings (especially fingertips), they can hurt a great deal. Luckily, healing is very quick because only the outermost layer of skin is affected.

You can tell these burns not only by the amount of howling the sufferer does when the accident occurs, but also by the resulting red skin. There will be no blisters on a first-degree burn, nor will the skin be broken. There may be some swelling on and around the burned area. This kind of burn affects only the outermost layers of the skin.

First-degree burns have slight redness or discoloration, along with a bit of swelling and pain.

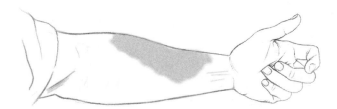

First-degree burns do not usually need professional medical attention. Simply cool the burn under cold, running water for several minutes to stop the burn from getting worse. You can give the injured person an aspirin (if he or she has no medical complications) and soothe the area with some aloe vera ointment or burn cream.

Second-Degree Burns

By the very nature of their place on the "burn hierarchy," these burns require some medical treatment. You can get a second-degree burn from too much sun, scalding hot soup, coffee, tea, or quick flash burns from gasoline or kerosene lamps.

Second-degree burns are distinguished by the blistery, red blotchy marks they leave on skin. Blisters form in these burns because the burn penetrates deeper into the layers of skin, releasing body fluids that erupt and cause blisters on the surface. Sometimes the burned area will swell or ooze, and it is painful.

Second-degree burns look red or mottled, and generally have blisters. These burns may ooze or swell.

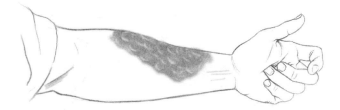

Pain from second-degree burns can be vastly reduced by preventing air from getting at those tender, exposed nerve endings and tissues. Here's the best emergency first aid, step-by-step:

1. Submerge the burned area in cold water (as cold as possible). If the burn occurred on the chest or back, pour cold water from a bucket or a hose directly onto the burn.

2. Keep the cold water on the burn until medical help arrives. If the burns are minor, keep them in cold water for at least five minutes.

3. If the burns are extensive, you can apply a cool, wet cloth to the affected area—but only if the dressing is wrapped in plastic. Cloth tends to adhere to burns, and it can worsen the pain if a physician has to pull it off to treat the burn.

4. If the burns are minor, you can treat them in the same way you'd treat first-degree ones. You won't need medical help. Simply pat the area dry and place a loose sterile cloth over it.

Burns in the Third Degree

Third-degree burns are serious—deadly serious. If you encounter someone who has a third-degree burn, get medical attention fast!

How do you know a third-degree burn from a first- or second-degree one? The injured person is literally burned, the skin is charred and white. All of the layers of skin are destroyed (sometimes quite obviously) with this kind of burn.

Third-degree burns come from situations like the ones you read about in the paper. Fireman rushing from burning buildings. People rolling on the ground with their clothes on fire. Pots of boiling water spilling on vulnerable skin. Accidents involving electrical outlets. Any of these can cause serious burns and shock.

> **First Things First**
> Did you know that third-degree burns hardly ever hurt at all, at least not initially? That's because nerve endings have been completely burned, and the brain hasn't yet received the painful message.

If the burned person shows any of the signs of shock, immediately treat that before taking care of the burn. See Chapter 3 for step-by-step instructions on treating shock.

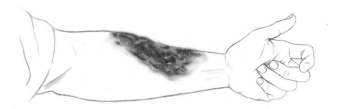

Third-degree burns look like deep wounds and often appear to be white and charred.

As we've already mentioned, third-degree burns are the most severe of all burns. They require medical treatment and precise first aid care. If you know what you are doing, you can help prevent infection from spreading.

1. Call for medical attention if access is immediately available.

2. Treat for shock, if necessary. This is especially true if the burn is caused by electric shock (see the last section of this chapter).

3. If you suspect chemical burning, especially from dangerous acids, you need to take first aid care one step further in order to stop the burn from spreading. As soon as you've called for medical help, pick up the phone and call the local poison control center. As with any type of poison ingestion or inhalation or burn, these specialists can tell you exactly what you need to do. (See Chapter 23 for more on poisoning.)

4. Remove any tight clothing or jewelry that's not on the actual burned area. With third-degree burns, there's always the danger of swelling which can cause blood vessels to constrict and create other complications.

5. You can submerge the burned area under cold running water, but avoid ice. Too much cold can exacerbate shock.

6. Pat the area dry and place a loose, sterile cloth over the area.

7. If hands are burned, elevate them, keeping them higher than the heart. This can be done by gently placing pillows under the injured person's arms.

8. Burned legs and feet should also be elevated to keep blood flowing smoothly.

9. Keep the injured person still. Do not let him or her walk around.

10. If the face is burned, keep checking for breathing complications. If airways seem to be blocked, follow the instructions Chapter 3 for performing mouth-to-mouth resuscitation.

11. Above all, get the burned victim to a hospital. Third-degree burn victims are prime candidates for infection, pneumonia, and other complications, and they need medical attention fast.

A Burn by Any Other Name

Whether the burn is caused by too many hours out in the sun, chemical acids, corrosives, or fire, the degree of burn is what counts—not the cause. Do keep in mind, however, that chemical burns are more complicated than those that result from fire. Certain acids need to be neutralized in order to prevent the burn from spreading and causing a lesser burn to develop into a third-degree burn. And, if you aren't sure where a burn fits in the "hierarchy," treat it as a third-degree burn. As the cliché says, it's better to be safe than sorry.

Dealing with Electric Shock

Electricity causes burns via the flow of electric voltage through the skin. But electric shock can cause more than burns. Bad shocks can cause deep tissue damage, and extremely high voltages may even stop the heart. You can tell an electric shock burn from other burns by the small, discolored marks on the skin at the electricity's entrance and exit locations.

The rest of this chapter deals with handling emergencies involving electric shocks, including steps to ensure your safety and help the injured person.

First, Turn Off the Power—If You Can

Before you can administer first aid to a person experiencing an electric shock, you must turn off the power. Don't waste time on appliance switches or plugs. Such things might have loose connections that could have caused the problem in the first place. The best solution? If you're in the house, immediately move to the master fuse and turn off all the power.

Sometimes the situations that cause electric shocks are very simple (such as dropping a hair dryer in the bathtub). However, they don't always occur in the kitchen or the bathroom. Sometimes a live wire can fall on a person outdoors, in which case there's no way to shut the power off. While you're waiting for help to arrive, there are a few things you can do to help—without injuring yourself.

> **Ouch!**
> Never try to pull a person away from the electrical current. If you do, you too will become a conductor; the current will run from that person's body into yours!

➤ Stand on a thick pile of newspapers or a fat rubber "welcome mat"—but only if the ground is not wet and it isn't raining. In such a case, the wetness would immediately make you a conductor regardless of what you're standing on.

➤ Using a wooden broom, mop, or pole, try to push the injured person off the live wire—or try to push the live wire off the injured person.

Always make sure the mat, the pole, and your hands are dry! The dry, insulated material you're standing on will prevent the electricity from flowing into you. When you've turned off the power source that caused the shock, or you have otherwise moved the power away from the injured person, you can help him or her to safety and get help.

Treating for Electric Shock Before Help Arrives

Before beginning first aid care, remember to call for emergency help and, as always, practice the universal safety guidelines discussed in Chapter 1.

1. Because shock is more of a risk with electricity than any other type of burn, check the injured person's ABCs and take the appropriate measures. (See the ABCs of first aid care in Chapter 1. They remind you to check Airways, Breathing, and Circulation.) If a person is not breathing, immediately begin mouth-to-mouth resuscitation as you learned in Chapter 3.

2. While waiting for help, apply a small amount of antibacterial or antiburn ointment on the points of entry and exit.

3. Keep the injured person on his or her back, with the feet and legs elevated.

4. If the injured person is unconscious, gently turn him or her to the side, supporting the head with a pillow. This will aid breathing and keep shock damage from increasing.

5. Gently cover the injured person with a blanket.

The Least You Need to Know

➤ Just because a bruise doesn't appear to be bleeding, doesn't mean that it isn't bleeding internally. Check for symptoms of internal bleeding (which resemble shock), and seek medical attention for the injured person if needed.

➤ Treating cuts, scrapes, bumps, and bruises depends on the intensity of the injury itself. Use ice to minimize swelling. In addition to that, keep bleeding to a minimum and cover the wound with a sterile, compact bandage.

➤ There are three types of burns: first-, second-, and third-degree. All three can be caused by fire, sun, or chemicals.

➤ When in doubt, treat all burns as if they are third-degree. Rinse the area with cold (not icy) water, keep it sterile, elevate extremities to inhibit blood flow and reduce swelling. Also, look for shock and seek medical help!

➤ All electric shock burns are third-degree burns. They can also stop the heart, so make sure Airways are clear, Breathing is present, and Circulation is good.

➤ Remember safety measures intended to protect yourself. Don't run into burning buildings. And don't try to pull an "electrified person" away before you turn off the power source!

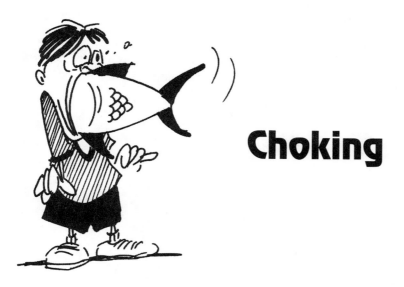

Chapter 9

Choking

In This Chapter

➤ Recognizing the signs of choking before it's too late

➤ Doing the Heimlich Maneuver

➤ Treating an infant who has swallowed something that's blocking the main airway

It happens so quickly. You are enjoying a nice dinner and without warning, your companion starts coughing. He or she turns red, and cannot talk. In short, this individual is choking. Or maybe you're at home, and a baby gets his or her hands on some pennies that just happen to look good enough to eat.

When a person is choking, he or she has a partially blocked or obstructed airway. In simple terms, that means he or she cannot breathe, and first aid must be administered fast!

This chapter shows you how to recognize when someone is choking. It also explains how to react under various conditions, such as when an infant is choking.

Signs and Symptoms of Choking

Choking can cause as much panic in the person observing the problem as in the person going through it. It is terrifying to watch someone who is unable to catch his or her breath. But you can't let the panic take over. First aid must be administered immediately.

Most of us can easily recognize the signs of choking:

Gasping for breath

Grabbing at the throat, mouth agape

Garbled, hoarse speaking

Clammy skin or sweating

Dizziness

Face turning red and tongue becoming swollen

Ultimately, unconsciousness

This is the universal sign for choking. Use it if you're choking; provide help if you see someone else using it.

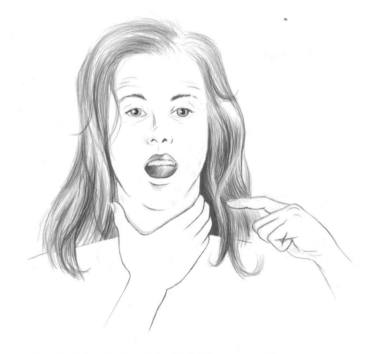

The most effective treatment for choking is the Heimlich Maneuver. If you or someone nearby demonstrates the universal sign for choking or shows any of the warning signals listed above, act quickly. Begin the Heimlich Maneuver, which you'll learn in the next section.

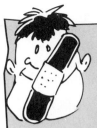

Before You Put the Band-Aid On

There are times when choking doesn't require the Heimlich Maneuver. If someone swallows a smooth object, no bigger than a marble or a coin, there can be signs of painful choking as the object passes down through the stomach and the esophagus (which is the smallest part of the digestive system). But as soon as the object passes through the esophagus and reaches the intestines, the fit of choking passes. Breathing is no longer obstructed, and eventually, the object will be passed. Do notify your physician, however, if someone swallows such an object, just to be sure there will be no aftereffects like infection or internal cuts.

Guide to the Heimlich Maneuver

Although it might sound like a military strategy, the Heimlich Maneuver is the creation of U.S. surgeon Henry J. Heimlich, M.D., whose simple and innovative technique became popular during the 1960s and is now required by law to be prominently displayed on a poster in public places.

The Heimlich Maneuver is a means of dislodging the food or object that is causing breathing problems. It involves hitting the back of an adult to loosen the object, and then applying pressure to the stomach.

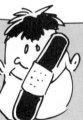

Before You Put the Band-Aid On

Dr. Henry J. Heimlich didn't wake up one morning and think up his famous maneuver. It took years of research and experience as a respiratory surgeon to design his simple technique—as well as to create other innovative procedures. Born in 1920 in Wilmington, Delaware, he was also an author and a professor of advanced clinical sciences at Xavier University in Cincinnati. He produced the films "How to Save a Choking Victim" (1976) and "Stress Relief: The Heimlich Method" (1983) and developed a unique operation for esophagus replacement using staples.

If someone is choking, ask him directly, "Are you choking?" If the person is crying, choking, or even wheezing out "I can't breathe," let him try to dislodge the object without intervention. A good, solid cough can do more than your manipulations.

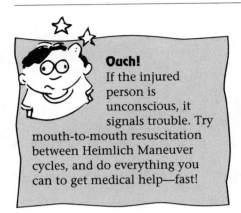

Ouch!
If the injured person is unconscious, it signals trouble. Try mouth-to-mouth resuscitation between Heimlich Maneuver cycles, and do everything you can to get medical help—fast!

Only use the Heimlich Maneuver if breathing has stopped or if the person cannot even call for help. However, if the person nods—if he cannot even talk or cough—call for help, and then follow these steps to perform the Heimlich maneuver.

1. Stand behind the choking victim.

2. Place one hand around the chest for support.

3. Lower his head.

4. Using the heel of your free hand, hit the victim's back hard, between the shoulder blades.

Try dislodging the object with blows to the back.

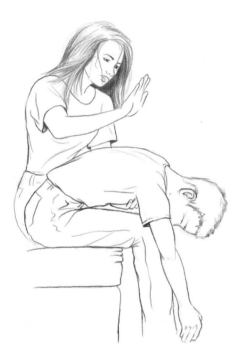

5. Repeat rapidly four times. This might be sufficient to dislodge the obstructing object. But if the person continues to choke, follow the remaining steps.

6. Put your arms around the injured person's torso, between the waist and the ribs, as shown in the far left drawing on the following page.

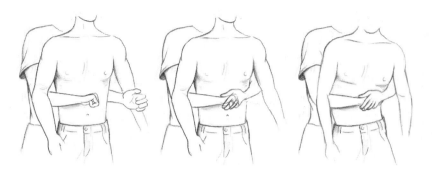

Wrap your arms around the person and apply pressure by thrusting in an inward and upward motion.

7. Place one hand with the thumb facing the stomach; with the other hand, grab the wrist of the first hand (as in the middle drawing).

8. Pull inward and upward hard four times in rapid succession (as in the rightmost drawing).

9. If the object is still lodged, don't give up! Repeat all eight steps until medical help arrives.

Special Heimlich Maneuvers for Special Situations

Infants can't tell you they can't breathe. But if they are coughing and crying, it's a good indication that they are not choking. Let them try to work the object out themselves, but be on guard.

If a baby's cough or cry is faint or nonexistent, first aid must be given. The Heimlich Maneuver is slightly different for infants under 18 months in trouble:

1. Before performing the Heimlich Maneuver, open the baby's mouth. If you can see the object that is causing the choking and you can reach it, perform the "finger sweep" to clean the mouth instead.

2. Place the baby face down on your forearm, your hand supporting the head (as shown in the first drawing below).

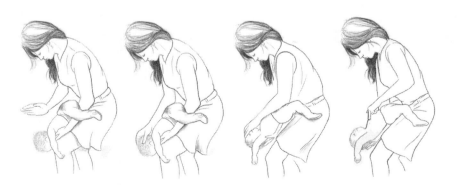

The Heimlich Maneuver for an infant.

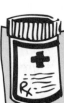

First Aids
The "finger sweep" is a technique that can be used if you can see the object causing the choking (in adults and children). If the person in trouble is not someone in your family, don protective gloves. Open the mouth and if you can see the object, literally sweep your fingers in the throat area, using feather-like, gentle movements to "rake" up the object and remove it. But *never* reach blindly into a choking victim's mouth. You can force the object down further!

3. Give the same four "hits" with the heel of your hand, but more gently, of course (see the second drawing)!

4. Turn the baby so he or she is facing you. Use both forearms and hold the head in the cup of your hand (see the third drawing).

5. Using only your fingertips, press down on the baby's chest four times (as shown in the fourth drawing).

6. Repeat the procedure until help comes.

Pregnant women and obese persons also need special care. The blows to the back remain the same, using the heel of the hand. However, when you put your arms around them for the forward thrusts, you must adapt to the excess weight. Instead of pressing your hands between the waist and ribs in the second part of the Maneuver, push your hands against the breastbone.

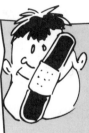

Before You Put the Band-Aid On

Breathing obstruction is usually associated with sleep apnea, of which snoring is a symptom. When you are asleep and breathing is obstructed, the throat relaxes as it should, but the tongue or some tissue on the throat itself obstructs the smooth passage of air. This situation can become serious if you try to get the air past the obstruction by inhaling harder, which is a reflex action. You can inhale so hard that the sides of the throat literally "clump together" and stick, like a hearty handshake. The result? The throat collapses completely, allowing *no* air to pass through. The result is a gasp, followed by a snore, followed by a gasp …and the cycle can continue. Eventually, a person *can* die of asphyxiation while sleeping!

Saving Yourself If You're Choking

What if *you* happen to be the person who chokes on a chicken bone, and there's no one around to help? Don't worry. The Heimlich Maneuver is so versatile, you can even perform it on yourself.

1. Dial the phone, knock on the wall, honk the horn, or anything to get help.

2. While you're waiting, lean over the back of a chair.

3. Push your stomach against the rim of the chair back as hard as you can.

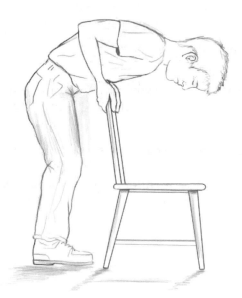

You can do the Heimlich Maneuver on yourself if you must.

Obstructions and Swallowed Objects

Swallowing small objects is usually not harmful. (Just ask any dog who's been left in the house alone!) Usually, there will be some discomfort as the object passes through the digestive tract, but, eventually, it will be expelled.

In certain circumstances, however, you should call for medical attention immediately. For example, if the swallowed object is sharp and dangerous, such as a pin, a sharp fish bone, a broken chicken bone, or an open safety pin. Likewise, you should seek help if the victim experiences excessive drooling or very severe pain that lasts longer than five minutes.

The Least You Need to Know

➤ Choking is one of the most common first aid situations. The universal sign for choking is to hold the throat and point to the mouth.

➤ Symptoms will pass if the person can talk, wheeze, cough, and especially scream.

➤ Practice the Heimlich Maneuver *before* you need it. As described in this chapter, start with sharp blows between the shoulder blades. Then clasp your hands in front of the victim's abdomen and pull in and up.

➤ The Maneuver is different for children under 18 months because you can cause damage to their tiny bodies if you perform it the way you do for adults.

➤ Pregnant women and obese people also need special, more effective care because of their excess weight.

➤ You can perform the Heimlich Maneuver on yourself by pressing your abdomen against the back of a chair and pushing. Of course, you should dial 911 before you start—just in case!

➤ Swallowing objects that are not potentially dangerous is usually okay. However, if someone swallows a sharp object, (a pin, a sharp bone, or a thumb tack, for example), he or she should seek medical attention. There is the danger of internal cuts and bleeding. And if an object is minuscule, an x-ray might have to be taken to find its exact location.

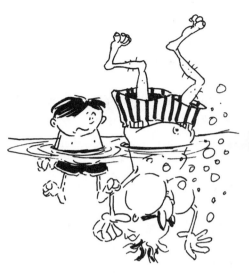

Drowning

Among accidental deaths in America, death by drowning is one of the most common causes. Drowning doesn't just happen in oceans, lakes, and through melting ice. You can drown in a bathtub—or even a wading pool.

Sometimes drowning occurs because of another injury, a heart attack or stroke that causes unconsciousness. Sometimes it can happen from a head injury caused by diving into shallow water. Cramps, too, can cause panic, which in turn may lead to drowning.

This chapter offers steps you can take to help rescue a drowning victim. It also provides the first aid steps to deal with the results of drowning, and to help resuscitate the victim.

Water Rescue

The signs for help are easy to identify. A cry, a splash by the arms and legs, and a period of immersion when the drowning victim disappears from sight are all signs that a person in the water may be drowning.

Rescue in a large body of water, unfortunately, is not quite as easy. But it is possible when the rescuer knows what he or she is doing:

1. If a lifeguard is nearby, let him or her do the rescuing! Otherwise, shout for help as loud as you can.

2. Try to reach the injured person without leaving the shore. Use your arm, your leg, a sweatshirt, life preserver, rope or rescue pole, or anything that can float.

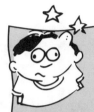

Ouch!
Oceans are vast places with strong currents and swirls. If you spot someone drowning far out in the water and you are on land, get help as fast as you can. As frustrating as it can be, the odds are against you. If you are not a lifeguard and equipped to handle crashing waves, you are likely to become a victim instead of a hero.

3. Hold onto something on solid ground (such as another person) with your other hand so you aren't swept away yourself by the strong currents.

4. If you can't reach the victim from the shore, locate a boat and find someone to assist you. Be sure that you, or someone with you, can operate the watercraft.

5. When a boat is not available, swim out to the spot where the victim was last seen—but only if you are a good swimmer. Currents, undertow, and cold water temperatures can hinder even average swimmers. Even if you are a good swimmer, always have a flotation device with you, something that the drowning victim can hold onto as you swim back to shore. If the drowning person is unconscious, you may have to hold the him or her on the flotation device as you return to shore using a side stroke and strong kicks.

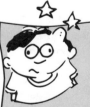

Ouch!
Never let a drowning person grab onto you in deep water. There's a chance that you will go under as well. If you are out of shape, don't even attempt to go out into the water. Your best bet is to call for help and be a landlubber hero.

Although the term "personal flotation device" might sound like some kind of politically correct euphemism, in reality, a flotation device such as a life preserver, life jacket, thick floating dinghy, or raft can save a life. All of these lightweight devices can keep a person afloat for a time and prevent him or her from drowning. Like the safety belts you wear when you drive, personal flotation devices are preventative devices. You should use one anytime you're out fishing, boating, or swimming far out at sea.

Reviving Someone Who Has Drowned or Swallowed Water

Suppose you manage to pull a drowning person back to dry land. What do you do next?

Rescue is only half the job. Reviving someone who has drowned or swallowed water is the other half, and it's equally important when it comes to saving a life.

Reviving a person involves performing mouth-to-mouth resuscitation (see Chapter 3). Of course, you should implement universal safety guidelines whenever possible. If you have an airway bag in your first aid kit, use it! It will provide safety during mouth-to-mouth resuscitation, keeping HIV and other infections at bay.

As always, call for help before beginning these important first aid emergency measures.

1. Turn the drowning person's head to the side, allowing any water to drain from his or her mouth and nose. Turn the head back to the center.

2. Begin mouth-to-mouth resuscitation on land, if possible, or in the water if the injured person needs immediate life-and-death measures. (See Chapter 3 for general resuscitation procedures.)

3. Strongly breathe four times into the mouth of the injured person as you pinch his or her nose, as shown in the following figure. This helps air get past any water that is clogging the breathing passageways and the lungs.

> **First Things First**
> Babies are particularly vulnerable to drowning incidents, even in wading pools because they sometimes don't have enough strength to pick up their heads. If you must perform mouth-to-mouth resuscitation on a baby, don't use forceful breaths. Instead, breathe gentle puffs of air into the baby's mouth and nose four times.

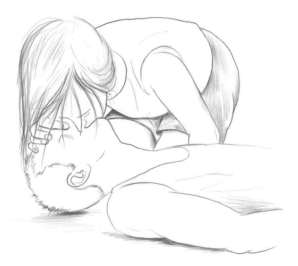

Mouth-to-mouth resuscitation for a drowning victim.

4. After four strong breaths, put your ear near the mouth and watch the chest for any breathing movement.

5. Check the pulse for signs of life.

6. Repeat the cycle.

Before You Put the Band-Aid On

Obviously, the chances of surviving from a near-drowning incident are much higher if the problem occurs when a person is in a pool than when he is in, say, the everglades or the ice slabs of Antarctica.

Hopefully, there is a lifeguard on duty, who is paying attention to what is going on in the water. If someone starts crying for help, or disappears in the water for more than a count of 10, it's time for fast action. When you get to the person, grab him around his upper torso, keeping his head above water. If the person resists as a result of fear and irrational panic, you might have to knock him out to safely carry him to the pool's edge. Be prepared to perform mouth-to-mouth resuscitation; don't forget your airway bag.

Here's a another special circumstance. Sometimes the water prevents good visibility. The solution? Goggles. There are even goggles that come equipped with waterproof flashlights or flashbulbs to help you find a victim. Look for air bubbles, water turbulence, or anything that looks like someone is struggling for breath.

You're not out of the water once the drowning victim starts to breathe and choke. In fact, the first 48 hours after a drowning incident can be the most dangerous. Complications resulting from water exposure—pneumonia, infection, heart failure—can all occur during this time. Therefore, you should always take a drowning victim to the hospital.

Ice Rescue

Ice fishing, skating, and snowmobiling are all dangerous sports because of the possibility of thin, weak ice. Without any warning, ice can crack, and you or your companion can fall through into the icy cold water. Two major concerns result. First, the water will be extremely cold and can cause severe hypothermia and frostbite. Second, the victim may become trapped underneath the ice and drown.

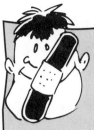

Before You Put the Band-Aid On

It's a cardinal rule: don't go ice fishing, ice skating, or crossing icy ponds by yourself. As is true in deep sea diving or swimming, the buddy system ensures you have someone to call for help just in case. But, if you happen to be alone and the worst happens, you can try to help yourself. Other people have done it, and so can you.

There are two main rules: 1) don't panic and 2) get out of the icy water as fast as possible. You will have a few minutes before hypothermia inhibits your intellect and your muscle function. Basically, you must crawl out of the ice. This can be tricky, especially if the ice above is thin and you can't get a good grasp or if the water currents are strong and determined to push you away from the opening. Don't waste time pulling off boots or coats, unless you can do so quickly and without tangling yourself. Dog paddle up and out of the ice, if you can, pushing out and over the ice with each arm movement.

Concentrate on getting out instead of on the scary thought of drowning. Panic can lead to hyperventilation, which will further inhibit breathing and circulation and can cause hypothermia to set in faster.

Ice rescue can be a challenge, but it is not impossible if you follow the rules presented next. As always, before beginning these "ice rescue" rules, call for professional help, either a nearby hospital, ambulance, or even a ranger. It's nice to know that backup is on its way while you proceed on "thin ice."

Rule #1: Don't step on the breaking ice yourself!

If you do, there will be two of you in need of help.

Rule #2: Reach for the person with a scarf or other clothing item, a tree limb, or a pole.

Using another object to reach the drowning person ensures that you keep your distance from the weak, dangerous ice. If there are others who can aid in the rescue attempt, you can form a human chain to reach the victim. To do so, each person lies face-down on firm ice and holds the ankles of the person in front of him. The "anchor man" should remain on shore, firmly gripping the legs of the first person lying down (and with a rope tied to his torso and a sturdy tree, if possible). The following drawing illustrates this procedure.

Use a human chain to rescue someone from the ice.

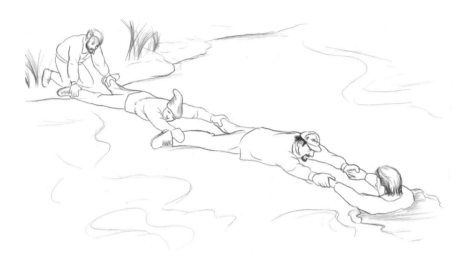

Another rescue device with "far-reaching" results is a small inflatable dinghy. Once blown up, it is smooth and sleek enough to get you across the ice to the victim, but light enough not to weigh you down. The dinghy can also be used as a life preserver, helping the victim reach up and out of the freezing water. But before you use any "hot air," make sure that the ice is strong enough to support your weight.

Rule #3: Slide the drowning person across the ice.

Never carry a victim across an icy body of water. The extra weight can make the ice crack, and then you're both submerged.

Rule #4: Begin mouth-to-mouth resuscitation.

Don't give up if the individual appears to be dead. Icy cold water lowers body temperature which, in turn, slows down all body functions. People have been known to be revived 20 minutes after a drowning incident with no brain or heart damage.

First Things First

Do not give up on a person if, after an hour's search on the ice, you still haven't found him or her. The frigid water slows down the body functions and what would drown a person in the tropics in five minutes can take over 60 minutes in freezing water!

Rule #5: Treat for shock if necessary.

Because of the frigid water, an injured person might be in shock. Cover him or her with a warm blanket to raise body temperature. Although it seems logical to give the person something hot to drink, you should *never* give food or drink to a person who's semi-conscious or who's suffering from shock. (See Chapter 3 for step-by-step instructions for treating shock.)

Rule #6: Treat for frostbite if necessary.

Frostbite is indicated by red skin, which then changes to a gray color, and ultimately changes to a bright icy whiteness (a sign of tissue damage). Treat frostbite by gently warming the body parts with lukewarm water. Do not massage the area. This can cause more tissue damage. Chapter 18 gives more details on treating hypothermia and frostbite.

Shock versus Hypothermia

Shock and hypothermia might sound like completely different conditions, but in many ways, they present the exact same symptoms and can lead to the same dire results. (See Chapter 3 for detailed first aid care for shock.)

Mild hypothermia occurs when the body's temperature drops below 98 degrees but remains above 90 degrees. Symptoms include:

Mumbled speech	Chills
Clumsy fine-hand movement	Lack of coordination
Skin numbness	Weakness
Shivering	Mild confusion

Severe hypothermia occurs when the body temperature drops below 90 degrees. Shivering might completely stop, but in its stead is paralysis, an irregular heartbeat, an inability to walk or stand, and eventually, unconsciousness that can lead to death.

If you think these symptoms sound like those of shock, you are right. Both can create intellectual, muscle, and heart dysfunction. Both can lead to death. The only difference is that shock occurs from a trauma to the body; it can occur in any climate. Hypothermia is directly related to body temperature and cold.

Treatment for hypothermia includes administering hot liquids, applying warm blankets to cover the entire body, and adding more heat piled up on the blankets. The key is to get the body temperature back up and to get the victim out of the "cold zone." Avoid the old tale about St. Bernard dogs and alcohol. Liquor can mess up body temperature regulation. You might think you are getting warm, but it's only a feeling, not reality.

Ouch!
Popular first aid treatment for hypothermia used to call for one vital element: an ambulance to get the victim to the hospital quickly. No more. Today, health professionals know that any form of movement can endanger the heart of a person suffering from hypothermia, creating dangerous heartbeat irregularities. Even emergency medical teams know to warm up the victim first. When they succeed in getting the temperature above 90 degrees, they move him or her to a hospital.

The Least You Need to Know

➤ Near drownings are among the more common accidents, but they don't have to end in tragedy.

➤ Never swim too far from shore and always call 911 first before you attempt any rescue!

➤ Know mouth-to-mouth resuscitation (see Chapter 3 for full details). After the rescue is complete, you will most likely need to resuscitate a near drowning victim.

➤ Never go on the ice to save someone unless you know the ice is strong enough to support you and a lightweight dinghy.

➤ Attempt to make a people chain if a person is far out across the ice.

➤ If you rescue a person who has been in icy waters, you must also treat for hypothermia, a condition in which the body temperature drops significantly.

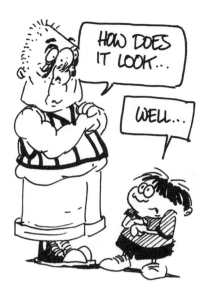

Chapter 11

Ear Aid, Eye Injuries, and Nose Damage

In This Chapter

➤ The best treatment for an earache

➤ Removing foreign objects from the ear without damaging the eardrum

➤ Removing an object from the eye

➤ Treating a black eye

➤ Stopping a nosebleed and treating a broken nose

The senses come alive at the sound of a familiar melody, the sight of your child's hair blowing in the wind, and the smell of a flower. The ears, eyes, and nose may give you access to the intense senses of smell, sight, and sound, but when they are damaged, they can give you intense pain. And injuries to these organs can be dangerous.

Knowing how to administer first aid to the ears, the eyes, and the nose can literally give back the sense of being alive. This chapter presents the first aid techniques for dealing with injuries to the ears, eyes, and nose.

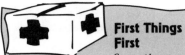

First Things First

Sometimes an ear injury can look worse than it really is. Profuse bleeding is not always a sign of something serious. Sometimes a lobe can be cut or the top of the ear may be nicked. Either way, a surface cut can cause a lot of bleeding, but it should be treated as only that: a cut. (To stop bleeding, follow the steps in Chapter 3.)

Ear Aid

Damage to the ear can be a signal of something more complicated or a problem all its own. If an ear is bleeding after a person has hit his or her head, immediate medical attention is necessary—especially if the person is unconscious (see Chapter 16, "Head Injury"). Otherwise, you should inspect the ear to look for the source of the bleeding and treat it accordingly.

Once you've ruled out simple cuts or head injuries, you can begin ear aid. First, understand that the ear is a rather complex organ. It has many delicate parts, which makes it subject to a number of different kinds of injuries. The following figure shows the various parts of the human ear.

There's more to the ear than meets the eye.

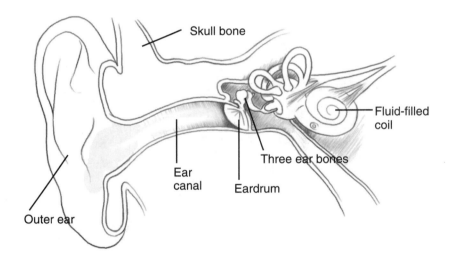

Six types of ear damage are possible:

> Swimmer's ear
>
> Water in the ear
>
> Earaches
>
> Foreign objects lodged in ear
>
> Pierced eardrum
>
> Loss of hearing

Because each of these problems requires special care, it pays to be able to identify the injury and provide the appropriate first aid. The next several pages explain how to handle problems of the ear.

Before you read on, though, understand that there are three "nevers" in ear first aid care. When you're helping someone with an ear injury, make sure you...

➤ never put anything inside a damaged ear.

➤ never try to stop the bleeding. This is one case when bleeding is encouraged. If you try to stop it, the blood can back up and seep into the inner ear. Stuffing cotton balls in the ear to clot fluids is a definite no-no!

➤ never shake, jiggle, or thump a person's head to restore hearing. Contrary to what some might think, people are not pinball machines.

Against the Tide: Swimmer's Ear

Contrary to popular belief, swimmer's ear—that uncomfortable, swollen feeling with the accompanying "swishing" sound—does not come from too much water in the ear or from eardrum damage caused by too much swimming. It is an inflammation or infection of the outer ear canal.

Swimmer's ear can be caused by bacteria or, like athlete's foot, it can also be a fungus. It becomes a problem when a person doesn't dry his or her ears well enough after a swim or when he or she stays in the water too long and the ear doesn't have time to dry. After the fact, the fungus grows in the ear. Swimmer's ear is never fatal, but medical attention is required. If left alone, swimmer's ear can cause infection and hearing loss. However, swimmer's ear is not an immediate emergency. A visit to the physician within one or two days can do the trick.

The main symptom of swimmer's ear is pain, possible swelling, redness, and itchiness. Over time, the ear can become clogged, resulting in a loss of hearing. There can also be a drainage of pus from the ear.

Swimmer's Ear Treatment "Strokes"

While you are waiting for your doctor's appointment, there are a few things you can do to ease the pain of swimmer's ear.

➤ Place a heating pad set to medium on the ear to help ease the soreness.

➤ Try to sit up as much as possible, even propping yourself up in bed with pillows. This allows blood to drain away from the ears so there's less "stuffiness."

➤ Drink lots of water and juice. Liquids not only help "flush" away infection, but the swallowing mechanism helps clear your ear canals.

➤ Chew gum. Chewing gum or food and yawning also help clear the ear canals and ease the pain.

➤ Take an over-the-counter anti-inflammatory medication such as Motrin or Advil. Tylenol, too, will help control the pain.

Water, Water Everywhere—Even in the Ear!

Things are not always what they seem, even in the cut-and-dry world of first aid. Water in the ear can cause the same symptoms as swimmer's ear, but in this case, there are no microorganisms playing havoc in your ear. Rather, water has actually gotten into the ear canal causing pain, redness, itchiness, swelling, and wax or pus build-up.

Water in the ear by itself is not a medical emergency. However, because it's difficult to differentiate between swimmer's ear and water in the ear, the best bet is to make sure the sufferer is comfortable and to seek medical attention within the next few days.

If the pain is intense, you can relieve pressure by following these steps:

1. Place a small drop of rubbing alcohol from your first aid kit into the ear.

2. Knead the lobe to make sure the water stays in.

3. Gently pat the ear and the surrounding area dry with a sterile cloth or cotton ball.

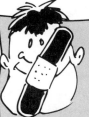

Before You Put the Band-Aid On

To avoid possible infection and wax build up, make sure you keep your ears clean. This means more than simply washing ears with a cloth when you're in the shower. To make sure ears are really clean and dry, use a cotton swab on the outer ridges and crevices of the ear. This prevents water from seeping into the ear and causing any type of infection. But never use a cotton swab in the inside of your ear, including the ear canal. It can damage an eardrum!

If you are having trouble hearing, it could be a simple case of wax build up, which can clog the ear passages. The best way to clean and remove wax is to buy an ear wash kit in the drug store. These kits are sold over-the-counter, complete with instructions, irrigation devices, and bulb syringes. They provide a means of safe, harmless, and effective wax cleaning.

The Beat That Goes On...and On: Pierced Eardrum

A pierced eardrum is more common than you might think. It can result from trying to clean the inside of the ear with a sharp object, pushing too hard with a cotton swab, a super loud noise, or a tear caused by a dive into a high pressure area.

The main symptom of a pierced eardrum is loss of hearing. If you or someone you're with experiences such a hearing loss, you should call for medical help immediately. And, as with any accident that pierces an organ or the skin, it hurts! In addition, you might also see some blood draining from the ear. If so, treat it in this way:

1. Cover the ear with a sterile gauze pad.

2. Tape the pad down loosely but securely.

3. Position the injured person on his or her side with the damaged ear toward the ground to encourage drainage. (Blood that pools in the ear can cause more hearing loss and possible infection.)

Listen to This! Earaches

Like tooth pain, an earache can consume the sufferer—especially if he or she is a young child. Remember the days when your mother or father had to put ear drops in your ears because you complained of pain? Then you would go to school and find that most of your classmates had a similar cotton ball stuffed in one ear.

Earaches are often the result of an isolated bacterial infection in the ear. They can stem from nasty head colds, which are viral infections kids can easily pick up from their classmates or on the playground (which explains why so many germ-prone children get them!). Sometimes they stem from a toothache or a jaw injury.

Although earaches are not usually immediate medical emergencies, they can be serious business. You should never treat them yourself. Take the individual to a doctor. Once the doctor determines the root of the problem, he or she can write a prescription for earache medicine, if necessary.

Ouch!
If you use ear drops every time someone complains of an earache, you can cause even more damage. If the earache is the result of a foreign object in the ear, the medicine might intensify the pain and spread the damage.

Of course, there's always the chance your physician can't see you until the next morning. So what do you do then? Especially if your child is crying out in pain?

101

Use lots of comforting sympathy.

Place a warm heating pad on the ear to soothe the pain.

Give an adult two Tylenol tablets; give a child Tylenol for kids.

Avoid getting the ear wet. Like colds, earaches are subdued by warmth. There's nothing bacteria likes better than cold, damp, dark places!

If you must shower, wear a cap to prevent water from getting into the ear.

I Can't Hear You!

Anytime one of the senses is "on the blink," the situation requires immediate attention. For example, loss of hearing can point to a much more serious audial condition, a head injury, or trauma. Because you're not a diagnostician, you should always make an appointment with your doctor if something seems out of whack. It's always better to be safe than sorry, and you should never feel foolish if the problem turns out to be simply an overload of wax.

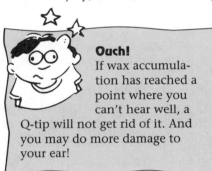

Ouch!
If wax accumulation has reached a point where you can't hear well, a Q-tip will not get rid of it. And you may do more damage to your ear!

Yes, loss of hearing can have a minor cause: accumulation of wax in the ear passage, which prevents the movement of sound vibrations traveling through the ear. There are special kits for removing wax from the ear, but you should check with your health professional before using one. A doctor can also perform wax removal in the office.

Foreign Objects in Foreign Places

Although it sounds crazy, an insect that's buzzing around can alight in a person's ear and become stuck. Unfortunately, it can easily happen to you, to a friend, or to your child. And insects are only one of the foreign objects that can literally fly into the ear. Anything in the air can potentially enter the ear and cause damage.

First Things First
If an insect flies into a person's ear, stay calm. If the insect is alive, it may buzz around and make an annoying sound. The individual may panic, scream, and shake his or her head to get rid of the noise. Although the feeling is disconcerting, it is not life-threatening. Remember the steps to follow in case of panic in an injured person (Chapter 4).

In addition to the things that end up in people's ears inadvertently, some things are put there intentionally. Many children have the delightful habit of testing out their nimble fingers and dexterity on tiny toys, jacks, beads, food, or coins and putting them compactly and complacently in their ear!

Here's a step-by-step guide to removing foreign objects from the ear.

1. If the object is a live insect, put a drop or two of mineral oil, baby oil, or vegetable oil in the ear canal. The oil will kill the insect.

2. If you can clearly see the object in the person's ear, carefully remove it with a pair of tweezers—but only if is near the surface.

3. If you cannot see the lodged object clearly or if it is lodged in the ear canal, tilt the sufferer's head to the side towards the injured ear.

4. Gently shake his or her head in this position.

5. If this doesn't work, leave the victim alone! Attempting to remove a deep or embedded object can damage the ear. Call for professional help.

> **First Aids**
> Even if you get the foreign object out of the ear, you should seek medical help. With an *otoscope* (an instrument that magnifies the eardrum), a professional can determine if all the material has been removed.

Eye Injuries

As I'm sure you well know, even an eyelash in your eye can be very painful. So an eye injury such as a black eye, a foreign object in the eye, or a cut on the cornea is definitely cause for medical attention.

Try to get in to see your family physician if that's possible. Your own physician is always your best bet because he or she knows you and your family—your medical history and medical insurance information doesn't have to be repeated.

Of course, as we all know, accidental injuries don't always take place at convenient times. If you can't see your family doctor, try a 24 hour Medicenter (a facility staffed with physicians for walk-in medical care). As a last resort, go to the hospital. Emergency rooms usually mean a long wait, but they are still your best bet if something happens in the middle of the night. Trust your judgment: If you are feeling panicked, take the injured person to the emergency room. However, if the situation seems to be under control and you are relatively calm, the Medicenter

> **First Aids**
> *Glaucoma* is a condition in which fluid builds up in the eye, creating pressure on the optic nerve in the back of the eye. It can result in blindness. Glaucoma usually builds slowly over time, and unfortunately, its early symptoms often are not noticed. Therefore, the best first aid medicine is prevention. You should visit your ophthalmologist or optician every two years to keep glaucoma at bay. Although rare, acute glaucoma (or, to be exact, *acute angle closure glaucoma*) causes immediate, sudden vision loss. Get thee to an emergency ward immediately if sudden vision loss occurs!

will probably suffice. (Sometimes the reason to go to the Medicenter or the emergency ward is one of convenience. Go to the one that is closer to your house!)

The main point is that you should get help quickly! Whether you go to your private physician, a Medicenter, or an emergency room, do not wait when someone suffers an injury to the eye.

There's a Fly in My Eye!

Flecks of dirt, bugs, and eyelashes all irritate the eye. Of course, they usually feel much bigger than they are: one grain of sand can feel like a large stone. In addition to pain and irritation, a foreign object in the eye can also cause redness, a stinging sensation when the person blinks, and sudden light sensitivity.

Unfortunately, these symptoms can cause someone to panic. An injured person's first impulse is usually to rub the eye to try to get rid of the pain. But this can have the opposite effect. Rubbing the eye can dig the dirt in deeper, causing more damage and making it even harder to remove.

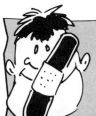

Ouch!
All foreign objects in the eye must be removed, but emergency medical aid is especially important if the injury affects the victim's vision. Specifically, if a person experiences blurred vision or sees waves, light specs, or blackness, he or she needs immediate attention.

Follow these instructions to remove an object that you can see from another person's eye:

1. Flush the eye with cool, clean water. Use a pitcher, a glass, or an eye dropper if you're not near a sink. If the object is lying on the surface of the eyeball, the flushing action should remove the object.

2. If you can still see the object on the eye and it does not flush out with the water, gently cover BOTH eyes with gauze pads and seek help as fast as you can.

Before You Put the Band-Aid On

Why cover both eyes if only one eye is affected? Your eyes work in combination. Keeping both eyes "closed" helps prevent all eye movement. This helps prevent excess irritation and provides a soothing effect (sort of a mini-sleep tank). Also, covering both eyes minimizes damage just in case there's an embedded object in the other eye that you cannot see.

If you cannot see anything in the injured person's eye, an object might be stuck under the eyelid. Follow these steps to treat that type of eye injury:

1. Flush the eye with cool, clean water and see if that alleviates the pain.

2. If flushing the eye doesn't work, first wash your hands to prevent infection.

3. Place the injured person under a good light (or anchor a flashlight so that you can see into the eye and still use both hands).

4. Have the person look up, and then you gently pull down the lower lid. If you can see a particle on the inside of the lower lid or at the lower edge of the eyeball, either flush it out with an eyedropper or gently touch a wet Q-tip or a moistened gauze strip or handkerchief to the particle so it adheres to the cotton.

5. Remove the Q-tip and rinse the eye with cool water.

6. If you can't see anything on the lower lid, check the upper one. Take another Q-tip and curl the lashes and upper lid over it. Be careful not to pull.

7. If you see an object on the upper lid or on the upper surface of the eyeball, try flushing it out with water while holding the curled Q-tip in place.

8. If that doesn't work, very gently touch the particle with a wet Q-tip to see if it will adhere to the cotton.

9. Release the upper lid and rinse the eye with cool water.

Ouch!
Removing an object with a Q-tip can be tricky. As with objects lodged in the ear, only use cotton swabs if you can see the particle on the eye's surface. If the particle doesn't stick to the Q-tip with a gentle touch, don't keep trying! You can cause more damage. Instead, cover the eyes with gauze pads and get medical help.

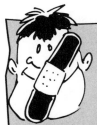

Before You Put the Band-Aid On

Although your eye does have a lid, eyelashes, and a continuous wash of fluid to keep infection and foreign objects at bay, sometimes that's still not enough. Shingles (a painful virus that is, in actuality, an adult form of chicken pox), Herpes Zoster (a virus that is a relative to the sexually-transmitted Herpes Complex), and poison ivy or other rashes don't always stay on the cheeks or eyelids. These conditions can get into the eye by way of rubbing or touching, and they can cause vision loss if not treated. If you or someone you love has an outbreak of any of these conditions, make sure to keep hands and hair away from the eye. And make sure you see your doctor for treatment of all the areas of your face, including the eye!

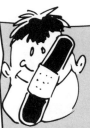

Before You Put the Band-Aid On

There's nothing rose-colored about "pink eye" (which is technically called conjunctivitis). It's a condition where thick, mucousy liquid drains from the eye, causing it to be "glued" shut, especially in the morning. (During the night you are in a prone position with your eyes shut; this makes the liquid "pool up.") Unfortunately, conjunctivitis, a bacterial infection, is easily passed from eye to eye and person to person. It is easily treated with drops or other medical therapy, so seek medical attention as quickly as you can. And, while you're waiting for the "pink eye" to disappear, keep your own counsel. In other words, use your own towels, pillow cases, and bedding. And throw out all of your old make-up! You can easily get "pink eye" again.

Eye Scream: Cuts & Scratches

Cuts to the eye are, well, obvious to the naked eye. A cut bleeds and causes distortion to the eyeball. But scratches are a different matter. They can be very subtle. A scratch might feel like a pebble (or more like a boulder to the person in question) that has gotten into the eye. It feels as if a foreign object has "flown in," even though you can't see anything. The eye can become bloodshot, and you might have trouble seeing clearly. Your eye will also feel very, very irritated.

Think of any cut or scratch on the eye as serious, and treat it as a medical emergency. Call for help, and while you are driving the injured person to a doctor, keep him or her in a semi-reclining position. Place a pillow beneath the head, if necessary. Cover both eyes with sterile gauze pads held in place with long strips of adhesive tape (as shown in the following illustration).

The list of DOs was easy. But just as important is the list of DON'Ts you need to follow when treating cuts or scratches on the eyeball, the eyelids, or even the skin around the eyes.

➤ Don't exert pressure on the eye to stop bleeding. Although it may look bad, eye bleeding is rarely dangerous, and pressure will only cause more damage to the delicate eye area.

➤ Don't attempt to remove contact lenses even if they are causing the injured person excessive pain. This too will exert pressure on the eye, which in turn can cause more damage.

➤ Don't let the injured person rub his or her eye. It will cause more irritation.

➤ Don't flush the eye with water. Bleeding, especially with loss of vision, can mean damage to the eyeball, a condition that water can further irritate.

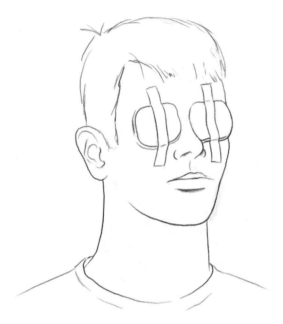

Covering and taping the eyes protects against further injury.

Contact Lens Problems

Many people wear contact lenses. A responsible ophthalmologist or optician will have you practice taking out and putting in your contact lenses when you first get them, and he or she will instruct you on the methods for keeping them sterile and clean.

Today, soft wear contacts are the most popular. They are flexible, easy to use, and unlikely to irritate the eye. (They also come in an array of fashion colors.) Hard lens contacts are more cumbersome, but they are more suitable for some eye conditions. And often, people who start with hard lenses tend to stay with them.

Choosing between hard and soft lenses is a matter of personal choice (like choosing between a stick shift

First Aids
An *ophthalmologist* is a medical doctor who specializes in diseases of the eye. Not only is she trained to examine eyes, but she is also capable of diagnosing and treating such conditions as astigmatism, glaucoma, and cataracts. An *optician* is also highly trained in examining eyes. He or she can fill an eyeglass prescription and provide contact lenses. If the optician notices peculiarities in the eye, he or she must refer the patient to an ophthalmologist.

and an automatic, a Mac and a PC, potato and potatoe). Regardless, most wearers become comfortable with the process of putting in and taking out within a few weeks. But contact lens accidents can still happen, no matter how long a person has worn them.

The most common problems that contact wearers face include:

➤ Hard lenses pop out. Surely you've seen people on their hands and knees searching the floor for a contact lens like it is the proverbial needle in a haystack. Missing lenses are hardly an emergency. However, it's always good to have an extra pair on hand when you're planning a trip.

➤ Wind, earth, and fire often irritate the eyes of contact wearers. So do mascara and other eye makeup. To prevent such irritations, you can keep the windows closed while driving in a car and wear non-prescription sunglasses for protection. You might also try using hypoallergenic cosmetics, going without mascara, and putting the contacts in after applying eyeliner and before applying mascara (if brush you must).

If a speck of dirt does get in the eye, there's no need to panic. Simply take out the contact, rewash in sterile solution, and then replace it. You might want to add rewetting drops if your eye is red and irritated.

➤ Pollen causes allergies to act up, resulting in itchy, watery eyes. If allergies are a problem, some people might have to go without contacts during the pollen season, and wear eyeglasses instead. If you are an allergic person but insist on wearing your contacts, make sure you drive in an air-conditioned car to prevent pollen from blowing into an open window. And always carry an extra lens case with you in case the irritation gets to be too much. You can also carry eye drops with you to soothe irritation.

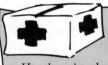

First Things First

Here's a simple tip just in case a dot of mascara or a fleck of dirt gets into your eye and, consequently, on to your contact lens. Always keep an extra contact lens case in your pocketbook, your attaché case, or even your back pocket. Make sure it's in fresh solution so that if you must take out your lens, you'll have a place to put it that's sterile and clean.

➤ A soft contact lens suddenly contracts, curling up into the top of the eye. This can be quite painful, but it is best not to panic. If possible, the wearer should gently move the upper lid over the contact, pushing the curled up lens to the side of the eye. With clean hands, he or she can then remove the lens. Always clean the contact before replacing it. To soothe red, irritated eyes (which result from all the poking and curling), place a few drops of eye drops or rewetting solution in your eyes and wait at least a half hour before replacing your lens.

➤ A contact gets stuck on the eye. Especially when a person first gets contacts, the contact will some-times adhere tightly to the eye. First, gently try to move it to the corner of the eye (as described in the previous item). If that doesn't work, have a medical professional take it out. You don't want to damage the eye. If it's the middle of the night and you can't get your contact out, try taking a few deep breaths (panicking won't help) and add rewetting solution to your eye to lubricate it. Then try again. If you still can't get your contact out, wait another 15 minutes. If you still have no luck, you'll have to go to the emergency room or a 24-hour Medicenter. Do not go to sleep with your contacts in (unless they are made for extended wear). Not only can that damage the eye, it can cause infection!

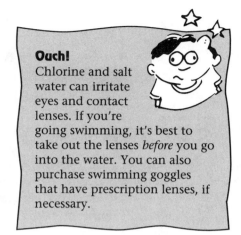

Ouch!
Chlorine and salt water can irritate eyes and contact lenses. If you're going swimming, it's best to take out the lenses *before* you go into the water. You can also purchase swimming goggles that have prescription lenses, if necessary.

Contact lens problems rarely call for emergency treatment. But, when combined with a black eye, a cut on the eye, or an embedded foreign object, they can signal danger. Follow the instructions for whichever specific eye emergency you're dealing with and keep contacts in place until help arrives.

Chemicals Get in Your Eyes

As discussed in Chapter 8, when a person comes into contact with certain chemicals, they can burn and cause damage to all areas of the body. Likewise, when some chemicals get in the eye, they can cause burns, terrible pain, and even blindness. Some of the chemicals that can burn the eye include:

Acid	Enzyme products used for clogged drains
Bleach	Bathroom and kitchen cleaners
Ammonia	Furniture oils
Hair dye	Alcohol

When a person gets a chemical in his eye, it is an emergency that requires immediate first aid. Follow these steps to administer the appropriate first aid treatment:

1. Tilt the injured person's head to the side toward the injured eye. (You don't want the chemicals to get in the good eye as well!)

2. Gently open the damaged eye the best that you can with the fingers of one hand.

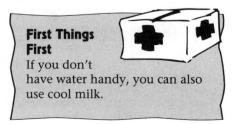

First Things First
If you don't have water handy, you can also use cool milk.

3. With the other hand, pour cool water into the eye.

4. Keep pouring water in the eye until help arrives. The more you flush the eye, the better the chances that the chemical will wash out and no permanent damage will be done.

A Black Eye

A black eye usually looks worse than it really is (emotional pain aside). Whether it's the result of a punch, walking into a wall, or extreme suction caused by tight goggles while swimming, a black eye needs medical attention. Sometimes there is bleeding that's not outwardly apparent. Likewise, the injury that caused the black eye may have also caused a contact lens to scratch the cornea. And if the black eye is accompanied by swelling, the swelling may affect a person's vision.

Sometimes a blow to the eye will cause swelling without "attractively colored hues." Treat swelling as you would discoloration. A bruise is a bruise is a bruise, whatever color it may be!

The best first aid is to take the injured person to a medical professional and let him or her take a look at the eye. While you're waiting:

1. Make sure the injured person is lying comfortably on his or her back.

2. Have the injured person keep his or her eyes shut. If necessary, cover both eyes with a sterile gauze pad. (When it is dark, there is less eye movement.)

3. Soak a washcloth, a gauze pad, or any available piece of cloth in cold water, and place the wet compress over the closed eyes to ease discomfort.

The Nose Knows: Nose Damage

We might not like its shape, and we might not like when it gets stuffed up. But, let's face it, without our noses we wouldn't be able to smell that fresh-baked bread, that just-bloomed rose, or that fabulous new perfume. And, as hearty as the nose might appear, it is made up of delicate cilia, or hairs, and sensitive tissue within the nasal cavities, which can bleed, bruise, and hurt if it is damaged in an accident.

Nosey Nosebleeds

Sure, if you hit someone in the nose, it's very possible the nose will bleed. But what about spontaneous nosebleeds—those sudden, worrisome bouts that seem to come from nowhere? Don't worry. In most cases, those seemingly unprovoked nosebleeds are more annoying than dangerous.

Technically, a nosebleed occurs when the tissue lining the inside of the nose becomes irritated. These irritations can be caused by any of the following things:

A dry nose caused by colds and sinus medicine

Excessive blowing from colds, flus, and allergies

Too much picking

Excessive use of nasal sprays

If someone around you suddenly gets a nosebleed, don't panic. Follow these steps for treatment:

1. If possible, have the injured person sit in a chair, leaning forward very slightly. (Leaning forward keeps blood from going down the throat and causing respiratory problems.)

2. Make sure the person doesn't swallow any blood; it can make him gag or vomit. Instead, ask him to spit out any blood that pools in the mouth.

3. Have the person apply pressure on the nostrils with the thumb and forefinger, pinching the nostrils tightly for at least 10 minutes. If the victim is too weak to do so, apply the pressure yourself (taking care to wear protective gloves).

4. While pinching, place a cold cloth on the nose. When the cloth begins to become warm, rewet it with more cold water.

5. After 10 minutes, slowly remove the fingers. If bleeding continues, roll two small pads of gauze to fit into each nostril. Insert them into the nose, making sure the ends of the gauze strips stick out for easy removal.

6. Pinch the nostrils again for another 10 minutes.

7. Remove the gauze pads.

8. If the person's nose is still bleeding, seek medical assistance.

Ouch!
Do not use cotton balls or band aids as pads for bleeding nostrils. They will stick to the inside of the nose and cause more irritation and bleeding.

A "Cauliflower" Nose

Ouch! A broken nose will usually cause severe pain, and in most cases, it will swell and appear to be bent peculiarly. Of course, sometimes a broken nose is not so obvious.

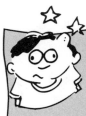

Ouch!
Broken noses heal fairly rapidly, but they can leave a person with a "cauliflower" nose. A deformed nose is not just a vanity issue: it can affect breathing and speaking. A reconstructive nose job will fix the problems caused by a broken nose, but it should not be performed until all swelling from the accident is gone.

Most of the time, when a person breaks her nose, she suffers a nosebleed. If someone has a nosebleed and you think the nose might be broken, treat the nosebleed (as described previously) and follow these additional steps:

1. Call for help. Medical intervention is necessary to reduce the amount of deformity and to ensure that there is no head injury.

2. Apply continuous cold compresses to the nose and face while you wait for help to arrive.

3. Keep the head tilted slightly forward.

4. Do not pack the nostrils with gauze. If a nose is broken, this can worsen the fracture.

Close Encounters of the Tiny Kind: Lodged Foreign Objects

Kids love their noses. They'll put anything in it: beads, toys, nuts, paper, raisins—you name it. Unfortunately, these foreign objects can become lodged in a nostril and cause pain and difficulty breathing.

If a foreign object gets stuck in your child's nose—or in an adult's nose, for that matter—you don't have to call for medical help immediately. Instead try these things:

1. Calm the child or adult down and ask him or her to breathe in and out through the mouth. Breathing through the nose will only irritate the condition.

2. Hold a tissue to the nose and ask the child or adult to blow the nose five to seven times.

3. If the object does not come out, seek medical help. Do *not* try to pull it out with tweezers or a Q-tip. You can cause damage to the inside of the nose.

The Least You Need to Know

➤ Do not automatically apply ointments or eardrops when a person has an earache. In fact, you should avoid these treatments!

➤ Excess wax can cause a loss of hearing. The wax builds up in the canal and acts as a "sound barrier." But don't use a Q-tip to clear up the excess. You can do more harm than good.

➤ You can kill a buzzing insect that's stuck in the ear by placing a drop of mineral oil in the ear canal.

➤ Black eyes are not usually serious—even though they hurt! However, they do require medical attention because there might be bleeding that's not noticeable on the surface. And, if it's combined with swelling, a black eye can affect your vision.

➤ Carry another pair of contacts (or a pair of glasses) with you in case of contact lens problems. Putting the contacts in a carrying case filled with lens solution ensures that the lenses remain sterile.

➤ Although bleeding from the eye does require medical attention, it often looks worse than it is. As with any cut, the bleeding must be staunched. A medical professional can best handle the problem to avoid any scratches to the cornea.

➤ Keep a person with a nosebleed or a bleeding, possibly broken nose in a sitting position leaning forward slightly. This will keep the bleeding from draining down the throat and might possibly staunch the flow.

➤ Never try to remove a foreign object from someone's nose by yourself. Even if you use tweezers and Q-tips, you can damage the nostrils because it's difficult to "see" what's up there.

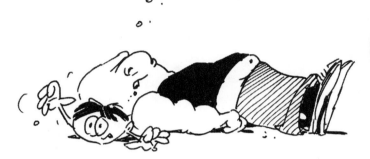

Fainting

In Victorian times, people (especially women) fainted all the time. It was considered feminine and was a sign of aristocratic good breeding. Today, however, we know that fainting is a signal that something is wrong inside the body. It can be a sign of danger to the heart or brain, a panic attack, hyperventilation (covered in detail in Chapter 7), malnutrition, or even pregnancy or menopause.

This chapter explains how to react and help when someone nearby faints (or passes out).

I Think I'm Going to Faint!: Warning Signs

The best news about fainting is that it usually doesn't occur suddenly. Often there are red flag signs that say, "Hey, I'm going to faint…." Of course, you have to be able to read the signs, which include the following:

Sudden paleness of the face

Cold, clammy skin

Dizziness

Nausea

Numbness or tingling in the fingers and toes

Sudden rapid or weak pulse

Feeling of panic

Blurred vision

If you notice these symptoms in someone nearby, immediately have him or her sit down and bend the head to the knees. If no chair is available, have the person lie down and elevate his or her legs approximately 12 inches.

If the fainting spell passes within 15 minutes, emergency medical attention is probably not necessary. However, fainting can signal a serious condition. Therefore, you should call your primary care physician and explain what happened, if only to put your mind at ease.

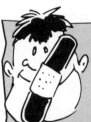

Before You Put the Band-Aid On

A full-fledged syncope, or fainting spell, is not normal during pregnancy. Blackouts and loss of consciousness are cause for concern if you are pregnant. Feeling faint, however, complete with low blood pressure and "falling out" (getting weak in the knees and going down) is quite common. If real fainting occurs during pregnancy, it's time to call the obstetrician. See Chapter 29 for details on this and other pregnancy emergencies.

Not for the Fainthearted: Treatment

Even if you know the signs, sometimes a person will faint before you can intervene. Don't panic. Here's a step-by-step guide for maintaining medical safety.

1. Lay the person down on the floor on his or her back.

2. Practice your ABCs of first aid (Chapter 1): make sure that the airways are clear, that the person is breathing, and that blood is circulating (listen for a heartbeat).

3. Loosen clothing if necessary to make sure the victim is comfortable and able to breathe clearly.

4. If you're inside a building, open the windows to allow air to circulate.

5. If the victim vomits while unconscious, turn his head to the side (or gently turn the patient completely on his side) and wipe out the mouth with a cloth.

6. Keep the chin up to prevent the victim's tongue from obstructing the throat.

7. Wipe the victim's face with a damp, cool cloth.

8. If the victim remains unconscious, or if he or she is conscious but is groggy, disoriented, and nauseated, it is best to call for medical help. If he or she regains consciousness, a phone call to the victim's primary care physician can dispel any doubts. If, however, fainting spells begin to occur frequently, seek help as quickly as possible.

Ouch!
If the person doesn't appear to be breathing or if his or her heartbeat is weak, immediately begin mouth-to-mouth resuscitation (see Chapter 3) and call for an ambulance.

Ouch!
Contrary to popular opinion, smelling salts should not be used when someone faints. In fact, administering smelling salts or giving the person liquid can cause him to choke and harm him even more.

Wake Up and Smell the Roses: Regaining Consciousness

When a person faints, he is rarely unconscious for long. Most people revive as they begin to fall down or after just a few minutes. As long as breathing and heartbeat are regular, the best thing for you to do is wait.

After the person regains consciousness, watch him or her for a few hours. The fainting spell can be a sign of an underlying, potential dangerous condition, such as dehydration, malnutrition, heart attack, stroke, or complications in pregnancy. You should be prepared for any contingency.

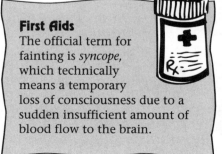

First Aids
The official term for fainting is *syncope*, which technically means a temporary loss of consciousness due to a sudden insufficient amount of blood flow to the brain.

The Crucial "Five Minutes" Rule

Suppose you are sitting in a chair, and the fainting victim is unconscious on the bed beside you. You've done your first aid steps, so you know that she is breathing and the heartbeat is sound. You wait …and wait….

If the person who fainted does not regain consciousness after five minutes, it's important that you seek emergency medical help immediately. A prolonged period of unconsciousness can mean serious underlying medical conditions.

The Least You Need to Know

➤ Fainting, in and of itself, is not usually an emergency condition. But it can signal an underlying problem, and if that problem goes untreated, fainting can create its own set of problems.

➤ Be aware of the signs that show the onset of fainting; they include clammy skin, dizziness, a pale face, and nausea.

➤ Follow the "five minutes" rule: If a person remains unconscious for more than five minutes, get help!

➤ Do not use smelling salts to revive someone.

➤ A person who has fainted should be placed in a prone position. Loosen his or her clothes and open nearby windows.

➤ Make sure airways are clear, breathing is regular, and circulation is normal (by listening to the heartbeat).

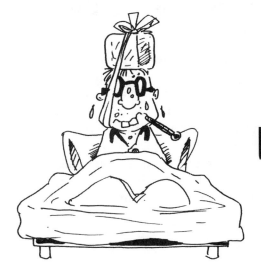

Fever

When a person has a fever, it is not an accident. It is not a sudden jolt from out of the blue. Fever is your body's way of telling you that something is wrong—that an infection has invaded your cells and that the antibodies of the immune system must go to work to neutralize the invading germs.

This chapter tells you how to avoid doing the wrong things when someone has a fever, and it tells you just exactly what you should do to ease the discomfort when someone has a fever.

Warning: Aspirin and Other Medications Can Be Hazardous to Your Health

Aspirin and other over-the-counter medications can work miracles on fever, cramps, aches, and pain. But remember to *always* read the specific warning labels on the medications you buy. Every medication has some kind of contraindication (warning of how it can be harmful). For example, antacids can be harmful if taken with certain antibiotics. Similarly, infants and young children who are given aspirin can come down with Reye's Syndrome, a potentially deadly disease which causes the blood pressure to rise and the brain to swell. Other medications can be harmful if you are taking high blood pressure medication, kidney medication, or antidepressants. If you are unsure about a certain over-the-counter medication, check with the pharmacist or your family physician.

You Give Me Fever: What Not to Do

Answer each of these statements with true or false:

You Give Me Fever

_____ Ice packs placed on the forehead will help reduce fever.

_____ A cold bath will lower a temperature quickly.

_____ Using alcohol in a sponge bath is more effective than plain water.

_____ Night-time liquids or syrups containing alcohol will help reduce the chills and pain of fever, as well as the fever itself.

_____ You should always take aspirin or acetaminophen (Tylenol) when you have a fever.

_____ Sweating will drive away a fever.

How did you fare? Did you answer true to any of these statements? Believe it or not, each and every one of them is false. And sometimes they can do more harm than good. Let's look at why you shouldn't do those things.

➤ Ice packs and cold baths can drop the body temperature too rapidly, and the fever sufferer can actually go into shock.

➤ Medicine that contains alcohol can throw off the body's natural thermostat. In some cases, the fever can actually get higher as a result.

➤ Sponge baths with a touch of alcohol are especially bad for babies. Alcohol can be absorbed through the skin, and it can harm an infant's vulnerable system.

➤ Although aspirin and acetaminophen do reduce fever, some people are allergic to aspirin or Tylenol. For people who are prone to bleeding or stomach upsets, aspirin can be very harmful. In addition, taking aspirin during the first trimester of pregnancy can cause fetal damage, and both can interfere with the immune system's natural response to infection. To be absolutely safe, check with your family physician before giving medication.

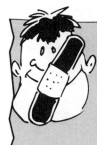

Before You Put the Band-Aid On

It's true that aspirin and acetaminophen can lessen the symptoms that usually accompany fever, as well as reduce fever itself. But follow the directions on the bottle explicitly, especially if the fever sufferer is a toddler or an infant.

➤ Contrary to popular belief, putting on an overcoat, a scarf, and a hat and bundling up under five down blankets will not break a fever.

Using a Thermometer

The most effective way to determine if someone has a fever is to take his or her temperature. Rectal thermometers are better for babies and people with colds who cannot breathe through their noses. Oral thermometers are acceptable for older children and adults. Note, however, that an oral thermometer only works correctly if the person has not had anything to eat or drink within the past half hour. If the person has had something, the thermometer is likely to give a false reading. Both oral and rectal thermometers are affected by exercise and hot baths or showers.

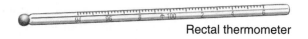
Rectal thermometer

Use a thermometer to gauge the severity of a fever.

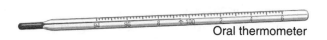
Oral thermometer

Follow these steps to take someone's temperature:

1. Make sure the person is well-rested so that the reading will be correct.

2. Wash the thermometer with lukewarm water and soap. Sterilize with a cotton ball soaked in alcohol. Wash off the alcohol with lukewarm water.

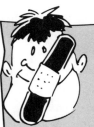

Before You Put the Band-Aid On

Today, there are lots of thermometers to choose from. There are disposable thermometers that you merely tear open and place in a person's mouth. There are digital thermometers that give even the most far-sighted person an easy-to-see reading. And hospitals use thermometers that you simply tuck under a patient's arm for a minute to get an accurate reading. Note, however, that you can't use an oral thermometer under the arm. Those "under the arm" thermometers are specifically designed to work with the body's makeup under your arm. Use an oral thermometer the way it is supposed to be used: in the mouth.

3. Shake the thermometer so the mercury inside will move past (below) 96–94 degrees. Hold the thermometer at the end opposite the metal bulb and shake hard from the wrist several times.

4. To use an oral thermometer, place the metal bulb of the thermometer in the mouth, diagonally under the tongue. Have the person close her mouth around the thermometer. Leave it in the mouth for five minutes. To use a rectal thermometer, dip the metal bulb in Vaseline for easier insertion. Gently insert the thermometer in the rectum approximately one inch in. Leave it in for three minutes, and wipe off the Vaseline before reading.

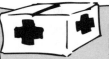

First Things First

Babies have a tendency to move around a lot, which makes it difficult to take their temperatures. Your best bet is to place the infant face down in your lap. Gently insert the rectal thermometer and hold your baby's buttocks in place for three minutes. Soothing sounds will help keep him or her from getting scared or restless.

5. To read the thermometer, hold the end opposite the metal bulb between your thumb and forefinger and turn the thermometer until you can see the sliver of color in the center. The number where the color stops is the temperature reading. Each line marks a degree, and even degree marks are numbered. An arrow usually points to the normal temperature: 98.6 degrees (see the following illustration).

Although "normal" temperature varies from person to person, the average is 98.6 degrees. However, temperatures can be lower in the morning and higher in the evening, and rectal thermometer readings are usually one or two degrees *higher* than oral readings.

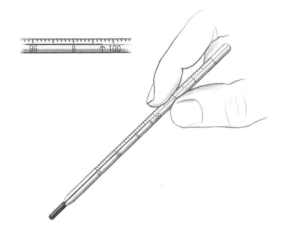

An arrow points to the "normal" temperature.

Treating Low-Grade Fever

If a person has a fever under 101 degrees, chances are he or she has only a mild infection. Make the person comfortable and have her take off any clothing (a coat or sweater, for example) that makes her hotter. The fever sufferer should not feel chilly, but she shouldn't feel like she's burning up either! Bed rest is the best medicine for mild fevers. Encourage the fever sufferer to drink plenty of non-alcoholic fluids (yes, the doctors are right about that one!). You might not have to call your doctor at all. Unless the fever lasts more than 48 hours or is accompanied by a rash, chills, or other symptoms, you can supply the cure: bed rest and fluids. If you do call your physician and he or she advises it, administer aspirin or Tylenol accordingly.

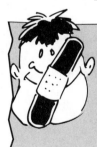

Before You Put the Band-Aid On

Water and fruit juices keep your body hydrated and help with toxic elimination. If diarrhea, vomiting, or a poor appetite is combined with the fever, water alone might be dangerous. Try alternating juice and water to maintain healthy blood sugar and blood salt levels.

Burning Up: High Fever First Aid

A fever higher than 101 degrees requires more finesse—and a bit more treatment. Although a high fever can still signal a minor flu or cold, it can also signify an underlying serious condition. When someone has a high fever, follow these steps:

1. Call your doctor immediately or seek medical help if you are away from home.

2. Administer Tylenol or aspirin as directed.

3. Give the person a "sitz" bath in a tub of lukewarm water. In a "sitz" bath, most of the person's body is exposed to the air and tepid water is poured over or sponged onto the body. This efficiently and effectively cools the body without causing adverse complications. If you are in a place where a tub is not handy, fill a basin, pitcher, or pail with tepid water. Pour the water with your hands or a sponge quickly over the fever sufferer's body.

4. Let the water evaporate into the air, but avoid any drafts.

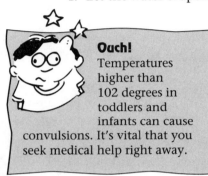

Ouch!
Temperatures higher than 102 degrees in toddlers and infants can cause convulsions. It's vital that you seek medical help right away.

5. Continue this process for half an hour unless the fever sufferer develops a chill.

6. Take his or her temperature again. If it's still high, repeat the sponge bath process for another 15 minutes.

7. Again, take his or her temperature. If it is still high, do not continue with the baths.

8. Rub the fever sufferer dry with a warm, dry towel and seek medical aid (at the doctor's office).

The Rash Connection

A red-colored rash or hives on the body along with a high fever often signals an allergy attack (see Chapter 7). If you or someone you're with experiences this, stop taking all medications immediately and get medical help as quickly as you can. But before you blame it on the medication, try to determine if the person has been bitten by an insect or if he or she has eaten something exotic. If you cannot pinpoint any other possible cause for the rash or hives, a medical professional can give you instructions on what to do next.

The Least You Need to Know

➤ Medical attention isn't needed unless a temperature is over 101 degrees.

➤ Old-fashioned remedies for reducing fever (including cold baths, cold compresses, and liquid medications containing alcohol) can actually make a fever worse!

➤ The only way to determine if a person has a fever is to take his temperature. Normal temperatures vary from individual to individual and from morning to night.

➤ A high fever requires special treatment—including a sitz bath and medical help.

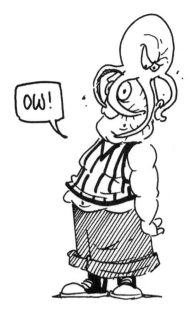

ow!

Fish Stings and Bites

In This Chapter

➤ Was it a jellyfish or a Portuguese man-of-war?

➤ Emergency first aid for shark or barracuda bites

➤ Which kinds of sea life are deadly—and which will watch you swim safely by

Thanks to the success of the movie *Jaws*, many people are not eager to just jump right in the ocean and swim out into the water. Although there's nothing like the serene blue water of the deep to calm the mind and soothe the spirit, a little knowledge is NOT a dangerous thing. When it comes to the oceans of the world, having a knowledge of sea life and being able to treat bites and stings can be more than helpful. It can save a life.

Because they are below and we are above, it's not always possible to determine what caused the sting. The best bet is to make sure there are no tentacles or tooth residue on the wound. Follow the directions in this chapter to treat marine life bites, and watch for danger signs such as shock, fever, and swelling. These require immediate medical help, whether you got them when swimming in the Great Salt Lake or Golden Pond.

In this chapter, imagine that you're a character from *Baywatch* (or any Peter Benchley novel, for that matter) and view the sea as they do: a world fraught with intrigue, danger, and adventure—especially from the marine life that calls the ocean home.

Jellyfish Stings

Jellyfish are aptly named. Their gelatinous, cloudy bodies look like globs of jelly. But the ugly body is not what's dangerous. The dangerous parts are the cells that adhere to their dangling brownish tentacles; those cells contain a poisonous and vicious venom that causes a painful sting in humans.

Jellyfish usually have a mushroom shape and a gel-like body.

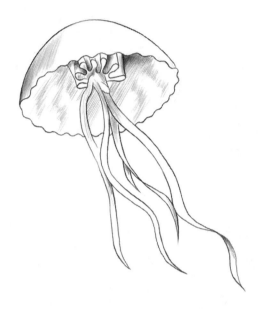

Jellyfish "epidemics" are usually cyclical, occurring at specific times during the summer. One day, you are swimming in clear water, and the next day the water is cloudy with floating jellyfish, adrift in the waves. Avoiding jellyfish is the best solution, but sometimes a long tentacle can get you even if the jellyfish body is far away. Symptoms of a jellyfish sting can include:

Immediate searing pain

Swelling at the sight

A red rash

Nausea and vomiting

Cramps

Shock (in severe cases)

Breathing problems (in severe cases)

If someone gets stung by a jellyfish, follow these steps to provide first aid for the wound:

1. Check vital signs. If the victim seems to be in shock or having trouble breathing, immediately begin first aid for these conditions (see Chapter 3) and call for medical help.

126

2. Wrapping your hand in a towel or wearing a protective glove, wipe away any dangling tentacles from the wound site. (Be careful. You don't want the tentacles to touch your skin!)

3. Remove any jewelry near the site (even from the hand/wrist if the upper arm is stung).

4. Alcohol or ammonia will neutralize a jellyfish's poison. Simply wash the wound with either one. Alcohol can be used full strength. However, you should dilute the ammonia with fresh water (1/4 part ammonia to 1 part fresh water). The chemical structure of salt water can dilute the ammonia's fighting power. If it's convenient, you can dilute a whole bottle of ammonia in two inches of bath water and have the victim sit in the bath for about an hour.

5. Dry the wound site with sand, powder, or cornstarch. Try not to apply creams or lotions if the sting is not neutralized because it might trap the poison in the skin.

> **Ouch!**
> It's always a good idea to have a physician check out fish bites, but not every bite is an emergency that requires *immediate* profession attention. If the person is suffering from shock, of course, help must be swift. Further, a sting on the face, especially near the eyes or the neck, can cause dangerous swelling, which should always receive quick medical attention. If you see signs of fever, swelling, or other atypical symptoms, get medical help. If there's nothing more than a painful sting, a topical antibacterial ointment and dressing might be all that's needed.

6. If there is swelling at the site, place a cold compress or an ice pack on the bite for twenty minutes every hour—or until help comes.

If the pain is very intense, try rinsing the bite site with some baking soda and water after you've followed your first aid steps. It can help decrease the pain until medical help arrives.

Even if the sting is mild and the victim feels fine soon after the episode, it's good to keep watch for up to three days later. Jellyfish stings can get infected days after the incident. The best prevention? Antibacterial ointment—once the stinging sensation is gone. Before then …ouch!

Portuguese Man-of-War Stings

They might not be politically correct, but Portuguese man-of-war don't seem to be the sort of marine life that would care. Found mainly in tropical seas, these creatures will burrow into the sand, hiding their brilliant blue bodies from probing eyes. Only their thin, dangling tentacles loll on the sand to be stepped on by bare, vulnerable feet.

A Portuguese man-of-war.

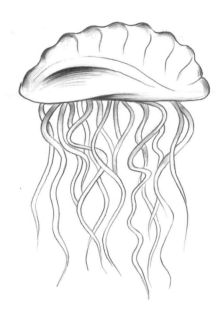

Portuguese man-of-war stings are very similar to jellyfish stings, and the symptoms are exactly the same. The good news is that ammonia or alcohol will also neutralize the toxic sting of the man-of-war. If you or someone around you suffers a man-of-war sting, quickly remove as many tentacles as you can and follow the treatment for jellyfish stings as outlined earlier.

Sea Urchins, Star Fish, Coral, and Sting Ray Stings

Ah, the mysterious marine life of the deep! The creatures are so beautiful to look at while snorkeling or scuba diving in the strange new land undersea. But looking and touching are two different things. As tempted as you may be, *never* pick up or touch marine life for safety's sake. Remember, curiosity killed the cat! And, unfortunately, many times, you can't be sure what exactly stung you while you were kicking up your heels in the galloping waves.

Here's an important rule: you'll know when you get bitten or stung. You'll feel the pain or see the blood.

Here's another rule: Always seek medical help for any marine life bite, especially if you don't know what bit you. To help you become familiar with some of the other creatures that you may encounter, see Table 14.1 and learn how to deal with resulting wounds.

Ouch!
If you go to the beach, sand is a fact of life. It might be a nuisance when you want to go home, but it also makes a great "towel" in an emergency. Sand won't cause an infection, and it will dry a wound when there's nothing else around.

Table 14.1 Other Toxic Forms of Sea Life

Object	Name	Object	Name
	Sea urchins		Sting rays
	Sea anemones		Fire coral
	Hydras		Cone shells

The Urchins of the Deep

Remember the "Tribbles" from the old *Star Trek* series? Those little spiky "golf-ball wannabe" creatures that quickly inhabited the Starship Enterprise? Well, sea urchins look very much like these tribbles—but they aren't quite as friendly. In fact, they're downright rude. A sea urchin doesn't actually seek you out to give you a mighty stick, but it does have deadly spikes. One wrong step and you can conceivably have a broken-off spike embedded in the sole of your foot! A sea urchin's sting can cause intense pain, swelling at the sting site, generalized weakness, and, in severe cases, paralysis.

A cone shell is only about three inches long. As its name implies, it looks like a cone with a wavy design. Like its sea urchin counterpart, it merely lies in wait until an unsuspecting swimmer steps on it. Its hard lines break the skin and release poison that seeps into your skin. It too can create nasty symptoms such as the following:

Intense pain

Numbness or tingling in the hands and feet

Problems breathing and swallowing

Blurred vision

Swelling at the bite site

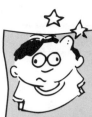

Ouch!
Never use this bandage method of "containment" on the neck, chest, or head. It can cause internal injury, including respiratory problems, loss of oxygen to the heart and brain, and possible sprains because of inept bandaging that keeps the body in an awkward position.

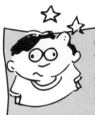

Ouch!
Tweezers might be great for removing mighty tentacles, but they are anathema to stingers. Pulling stingers out of the skin with tweezers can actually squeeze more venom into the system! And this also goes for spikes, which usually have a deadly barbed twist to them! Again, if you can, wait for help to arrive before trying to pry anything out.

Always call for medical attention anytime someone gets a "mysterious" marine life bite. And, while you're waiting, use the following first aid steps to minimize discomfort and injury. These steps are also useful for sea urchin and cone shell injuries:

1. Ask the injured person to lie down, keeping the bite or sting site still and positioned lower than the heart (to avoid circulating the toxins).

2. As with snake bites (Chapter 6), a snug bandage two to four inches above the site will help keep the toxins localized. Use a strip of clothing, a belt, or even a watchband to make your bandage. Twirl it around the leg or arm and tie it in a knot. Make sure you can fit a finger underneath the bandage.

3. If the swelling increases up to the bandage line, add another bandage two to four inches higher than the first.

4. Remove the first bandage.

5. Using a towel or protective gloves, get rid of any tentacles at the bite site. (Tweezers work well, as long as you are wearing gloves.)

6. Stingers and spikes need to be treated more carefully. If help is on the way and the stinger or spike is deeply embedded, you should leave it where it is. Spikes can be especially difficult to remove because they are often barbed. Trying to "pry" out a stinger or spike can make ugly wounds uglier. But, if help is not anywhere near, you'll have no choice. Use the edge of a clean knife or razor blade and slowly move the blade upward, lifting and "prying" the stinger out (see the following illustration).

7. Wash the bite site with soap and water to avoid infection.

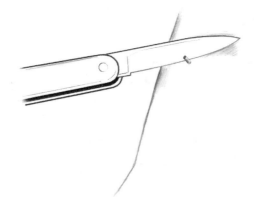

Use a knife to "pry" out a stinger by lifting it up.

The Mysterious Marine Life That Looks Like a Plant—But Is Very Much Alive

Sea anemones and hydras might look like beautiful, exotic plants, but, in reality, they are dangerous. Both these flower-like creatures, with tentacles that languidly move in the water, have one major handicap: They cannot move.

Unfortunately, you or someone you know can step on one or temptingly touch their tentacle flowers. As with all marine life, symptoms for injuries from both creatures include intense, burning pain plus chills, cramps, and diarrhea. Luckily, the toxin in tentacles is milder than the poison found in urchins and cone shells.

Treating the stings of sea anemones and hydras is relatively easy. Heat will neutralize any toxins, so simply soak the bite site in a pail of water that is as hot as the injured person can handle (without burning or scalding). Add hot water as it cools, and keep it soaking for at least thirty minutes to an hour—or until help arrives.

Marine Life That Looks Like an Inanimate Stone in a Meditative Garden

The fiery red beauty of coral is beautiful to even the most unenthusiastic ocean traveler. Unfortunately, not every coral reef you encounter is safe to climb, touch, and handle. And some coral is alive, harsh, and poisonous. (In addition, physical contact to a reef can cause ecological danger!)

Fire coral is particularly nasty. Its "cute" clusters of stout, short branches make it look harmless, but, in reality, its touch is worse than 100 fire ants. The main

Ouch!
Never touch, walk on, climb, or collect *any* type of coral. The slightest activity can do irreparable harm to the delicate ecosystem. If you do come into contact with coral, it should be because of an accident only!

symptom of this coral's "sting," caused by the slightest touch of its toxic surface, is a terrible burning sensation at the wound site.

The only treatment you can administer for contact with fire coral is to wash the area with soap and water and keep it clean until help arrives. Stay with the injured person to ensure that he or she does not go into shock. (See Chapter 3 for more about treating shock.)

The wound site might be bleeding—which will help eliminate any toxins. However, the bleeding can be so profuse that you will have to follow the steps for stopping bleeding (see Chapter 3) by applying direct pressure at the site. Just walking on a reef or on any coral can create a set of cuts and scrapes—all of which will bleed and need to be treated accordingly.

Identifying Sting Rays Is Easy

A sting ray is a creature that looks a little like a flying saucer or kite: it has a flat, blade-like body and a long, sinewy tail. You can see a sting ray coming—and you will know when it strikes. Symptoms of a sting ray injury can include:

First Aids
A *skate* is a creature that looks like a sting ray. In fact, they are related. Some skates like to doze on the ocean floor. They are soon covered and camouflaged with sand. As soon as someone steps on a skate, it reacts!

Intense pain	Sweating
Clammy skin	Nausea
Dizziness and weakness	Eventual paralysis and shock

The sting ray's sting site is pale at first, and then it slowly turns a bright red. It "stings" with a spike or barb that's located on its fast tail. But however the wound is inflicted, it is serious business, especially if the barbs on the tail's spine (which, incidentally, grow back!) are embedded in the skin. Call for medical help immediately, and then follow this treatment regimen:

1. Try to remove as many "stingers" as possible from the bite site, using a towel as "exfoliation" or a set of tweezers to pick at the wound site. Wear protective gloves to avoid contamination. If material is embedded, surgery might be necessary.

2. Sting ray toxins, like fire coral, are neutralized by heat. Thus, soak the bite site in water that is as hot as the injured person can stand.

3. Wipe away any blood with a clean towel. Apply pressure if bleeding is profuse.

4. Cover the injured person with a warm blanket. Shock is a greater risk with string ray bites than with fire coral. Be ever vigilant of the injured person's breathing until help arrives on the scene. (See Chapter 3 for information about treating shock and performing mouth-to-mouth resuscitation.)

Emergency Aid for Shark and Barracuda Bites

Obviously, a shark or barracuda bite can be life-threatening and help must be called immediately. Hopefully, a lifeguard trained in CPR can help restore breathing, if needed, while you wait for an emergency medical team to arrive.

In the event that you must handle the situation alone, there are steps you can take:

1. Call for help—immediately.

2. Help the injured person out of the water, if possible (see Chapter 10 for more about water rescue). But be careful: if you enter the water during an attack, you can be the next victim!

3. If bites are large and are located in the abdominal cavity, do *not* try to put body organs back. You'll only cause more damage. Gently cover the wound and organs with material that will not stick, such as foil, a moistened cloth, or plastic wrap.

4. If bites open the chest wall, make an airtight bandage with non-stick materials, such as foil, plastic wrap, gauze pads, or towels.

   Ask the injured person to exhale. Tape the wound completely and thoroughly as he or she breathes out. Adhesive bandages or even a belt will work.

   Keep head and shoulders up.

5. If a bite is deep, the most crucial step is to stop bleeding and treat for shock (see Chapter 3). Place a blanket over the injured person. Try to stay calm and try to soothe the injured person. Get help as fast as you can.

6. If a bite dismembers a finger, a toe, an arm, or a leg and you can find it, carefully wrap the detached body part in a sealed plastic bag, place it on ice in a cooler, if possible, and send it to the hospital with the medical professionals that arrive. It is possible that the body part can be reattached.

Shark and barracuda bites are dangerous. Unfortunately, while many have lived through the agony of a bite, many others have died. The best advice? Heed the warnings of lifeguards. Don't go near the water if there is a shark warning out. Don't swim in unfamiliar, isolated waters, especially in areas known to breed sharks and barracudas. And *never* swim alone.

The Least You Need to Know

➤ Jellyfish and Portuguese man-of-war toxins are neutralized by ammonia mixed with water or alcohol.

➤ Do not use salt water to clean jellyfish wounds. It can create more pain. Instead try to use fresh water mixed with ammonia or plain alcohol.

➤ Heat can neutralize the toxins in sting rays, sea anemones, and hydras. Soak wounds from these creatures in water as hot as the injured person can stand that doesn't cause scalding or burns.

➤ Coral can cause a fiery, burning pain, and its rough surface can create cuts and bruises that have nothing to do with the actual sting.

➤ Sharks can kill. Stay out of water that has shark or barracuda warnings! If injury occurs, contain bleeding, treat for shock, and call for help.

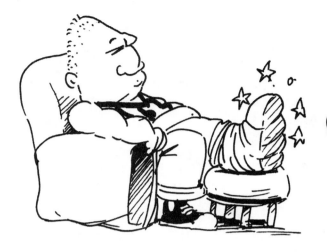

Gout Bout

If you've ever had a gout attack, you're in good company. Kings and queens, including the famous Henry VIII, often suffered from gout. Gout is a disease that used to be proudly borne by aristocracy as a "result of the good life," because of its onset after years of heavy drinking and even heavier eating. Today, gout is no longer mistaken as a disease that strictly results from lifestyle. Any adult, at any age, can get gout. And although the condition has to do with a build up of chemicals in the body, it is more a result of a malfunction in the body than it is from years of too many beers.

Whatever your attitude about gout, when it attacks, it comes on fast and furious—and it can ruin a fabulous vacation, an important business meeting, or even a good night's sleep if you're not prepared. This chapter explains how you can learn to recognize and deal with gout when it occurs.

Recognizing the Signs

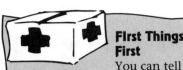

First Things First
You can tell the difference between gout and other inflammatory conditions, such as arthritis, by its acute sudden attack without trauma. Arthritis and other muscle pain comes on slowly, building up over a period of time. But gout hits fast—especially in the fingers and toes.

Gout is caused by too much uric acid within the body. As uric acid builds up in the system, it creates uric acid crystals, which are deposited in the joints—especially the big toe. These deposits make the joints swell, forcing tissue to "push" against the nerve endings. This eventually creates the pain called gout.

Symptoms of gout include:

Acutely swollen, tender area (that has not been the site of trauma)

Acute throbbing sensation

Pain when using the afflicted joint (such as taking a step on that big toe)

Fever

Chills

Easing the Pain

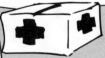

First Things First
Check with your physician before you take any medication. Gout medicine can cause such side-effects as stomach pain, diarrhea, and digestive problems. In addition, it can have dangerous side effects when taken with certain high blood pressure medication.

If you have one gout attack, chances are you'll have another. Therefore, you should see your family physician for help. A physician can prescribe anti-inflammatory medication to help lessen the discomfort, as well as a daily medication to control the level of uric acid in the body—and help you avoid another attack.

If you're planning to go out of town, it's a good idea to take a few painkillers with you, just in case. The best over-the-counter medication for treating pain associated with gout is ibuprofen (the generic name for the medication found in Advil and Nuprin). It reduces the inflammation of the joints, which causes the pinching of the nerves.

Administering first aid treatment is not an emergency, unless the patient also suffers from a heart ailment. Keeping the gout sufferer off of his or her feet for a few days and keeping the foot raised and "shoeless" is about the best you can do—along with administering anti-inflammatory medication as directed by a physician to decrease the irritation and inflammation in the joint.

Prevention Is the Best Medicine

Gout can be avoided—and not just by taking medication to control the acid. You can take the following preventative measures right now to avoid gout later:

➤ If you are obese, lose weight—but do so gradually. Quick weight loss fixes can actually precipitate an attack.

➤ Avoid foods rich in proteins that break down into uric acid, such as shellfish, deli and smoked meats, sardines, yeast, asparagus, mushrooms, and anchovies.

➤ Reduce your alcohol intake. Alcohol is two-fold trouble: it increases the production of uric acid as it reduces the body's ability to eliminate it.

Ouch!
Taking aspirin for gout is not a good idea. It can actually make the condition worse because aspirin inhibits the body's ability to eliminate uric acid. Likewise, acetaminophen is ineffective for treating gout; you might as well take a few stoic deep breaths instead.

➤ Drink plenty of fluids, especially water. The more you drink, the more you will urinate and the more uric acid (a gout catalyst) that will be eliminated. People with gout usually don't eliminate enough uric acid in their urine; they always have the same fixed amount of uric acid per liter of urine. However, the more they urinate, the more of that "fixed" amount that will be eliminated, too!

➤ Try stress-reducing exercises, such as meditation, deep breathing, or stretching.

➤ Limit your intake of Vitamin A to no more than 5,000mg per day, and limit your Niacin intake to only 100mg per day.

➤ Increase fiber in your diet by adding raw fruits and vegetables to your meals.

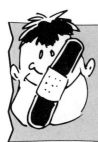

Before You Put the Band-Aid On

Beta Carotene is a better and more natural source for Vitamin A than a multi-vitamin or a Vitamin A capsule. You get it in carrots, mangoes, winter squash, kale, spinach, and cantaloupe.

As odd as it seems, studies show that eating a handful of cherries every day can prevent gout. The substances found in cherries and other dark berries keep collagen from breaking down, thereby inhibiting the formation of uric acid. And as a bonus, it also has anti-aging characteristics!

The Least You Need to Know

➤ Although gout is not a life-threatening emergency, it can cause terrible pain. (And it can ruin a long-awaited vacation or make routine days a terrible drudgery!)

➤ Gout is the result of a build up of uric acid in the body. The uric acid creates crystal deposits that tend to make for big, round toes!

➤ Ibuprofen and prescription medicine can eliminate the pain of gout and prevent recurrences. You should always check with your physician before taking medication.

➤ Resting and elevating the affected extremity are two easy ways to lessen the effects of gout.

➤ You can help prevent gout by eating right, avoiding stress, and drinking plenty of fluids.

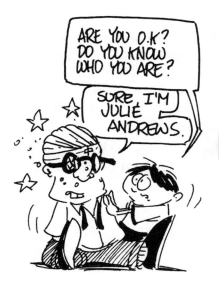

Head Injury

More than 500,000 people suffer from head injuries every day, most of which are the result of car, bike, and motorcycle accidents and falls. Because today's technology is so advanced, people who would have once been pronounced DOA due to head injuries are now able to live functional, full lives. But that's only possible if a person receives help right away and begins rehabilitation quickly.

It's not always possible to tell if a person has a head injury. Most are closed injuries; therefore, skull fractures and bleeding are not present. Making things even more complicated is the fact that the brain rarely works alone. The spinal cord can also be affected to a lesser or stronger degree. For example, when Christopher Reeves fell off his horse, he suffered a spinal injury that hurt his ability to even breathe by himself. Mr. Reeves' condition exemplifies what is so serious—and traumatic—about head injury.

In this chapter, we will first identify the areas of the brain so you can understand the serious dynamics of head injury. We will then describe the different types of injury and how to treat them.

Why Head Injuries Are So Dangerous

There's no disputing the fact that a bump on the head is much different than a bump on the knee, and that the bump on the head produces broader implications for long-term health. Depending on what part of the head is injured (and, therefore, the passageways in the brain that are damaged), the injured person can lose the ability to speak or walk or even remember his name. The brain, after all, regulates all body functions. It tells us what to think and what to feel, and it is what makes us human—and unique.

There are six distinct areas of the brain (see the following figure). Each of those areas controls different body functions that can be affected or disabled as the result of a head injury.

The parts of the brain.

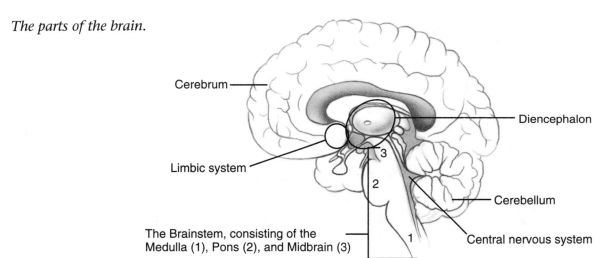

Cerebrum

Diencephalon

Limbic system

Cerebellum

The Brainstem, consisting of the
Medulla (1), Pons (2), and Midbrain (3)

Central nervous system

This list looks at each of the different parts of the brain in detail and outlines the function of each—which can be affected if that part is accidentally damaged. It will help you understand what's going on if a head injury occurs.

➤ **CNS** No, it's not a new bank. The CNS is the central nervous system, and it functions as the go-between that sends messages back and forth from the masses of peripheral nerves in the body to the spinal cord that leads to the brain. Damage here can affect a person's ability to move.

➤ **Brainstem** You'll find the brainstem at the uppermost tip of the spinal cord. Connected to the spinal cord by thick nerve fibers, it's the invisible underbelly of the "corporation." It is divided into three areas: the Medulla is the place where basic life functions such as heartbeat, temperature, and breathing are regulated. Moving up the brainstem, we next come to the Pons: the bridge between the medulla and the "upper echelons" of the brain. It is also the area where reflexes are controlled and instinctively used, and it houses the brain's alarm nerve cells that keep you alert. The third area of the brainstem is the Midbrain, which provides eye muscle control, as well as helping the Pons with its basic job.

➤ **Cerebellum**   Located behind the brainstem, the cerebellum is the body's center for balance and coordination: every step and every movement is regulated from here. The cerebellum acts as a traffic coordinator of your body's corporation, too. It coordinates your movement and your speech muscles.

➤ **Diencephalon**   Considered the "outer corridor" of mind power, the diencephalon sits above the brainstem, as a proud, majestic gateway to the emotional and mental depth above. Here, the hypothalamus and the thalamus—the partners in crime—decipher every sensation. These two partners also delegate where memory will be stored.

The thalamus is a beehive of activity through which messages are transported to the place that determines who gets what in the "upper echelons" of power. To illustrate its function, think of this. The words of the poem you're reading sit next to your recipe for veggie burgers in your memory storage tank. The words of the poem are sent to both the emotional core of the brain (where they affect your feelings) and the intellectual center of the brain (where they are deciphered and analyzed). They bounce from emotion to intellect and evoke the deep sigh you produce. In the meantime, the smell of those cooking veggie burgers is sent to the brainstem, which activates your salivary glands in anticipation of lunch. All this and more. The thalamus never stops!

The hypothalamus, though no bigger than a pea, is also a whirling dynamo. It controls basic instincts ranging from appetite to sexual arousal and from thirst to sleep. Thanks to its position close to the pituitary gland—the master gland of the body—it also controls the hormonal (chemical) secretions that, as they propel messages through the brain, determine the underlying basis of what we are, how we feel, and what we think, as well as "telling" the pituitary gland which hormones to release for growth, metabolism, sex, lactation, and other

First Aids
Short-term memory enables you to remember things about this morning or the movie you saw at the mall last week. *Long-term memory* accounts for those deep-seated remembrances of long-ago birthday parties, old friends, and music to which you once danced the night away. It also "locks in" repetitious, rote-learned motor skills, such as how to tie your shoe. The two types of memories are kept in "chemical loops" in different parts of the brain. Because short-term memory is stored in an area that's vulnerable to head injury and it has not yet become ingrained in the brain by repetition, it is usually more affected from an accident.

"basics." Because it lies so close to the "upper crust" of the brain, it also helps regulate our emotions, motivations, and moods.

➤ **Limbic System** This region, located between the Diencephalon and the intellectual Cerebrum, packs a big whallop in the human experience. We can experience joy, anger, happiness, fear, and many variations of those. Thanks to this area of the brain, our emotions get dimension and feelings—the color and depth that makes life a celebration. Together with the intellect, the Limbic System deciphers the messages it receives from below and creates emotional responses to them.

➤ **Cerebrum** You might call it the CEO, the Man, or the Head Honcho. The cerebrum is the intellectual heart of the very being. Here, the higher functions decode and respond to the various messages coming in from the areas of memory, thought, and even emotion. This part of the brain enables you to understand and organize your thoughts, to perceive the world and its meaning, to communicate, to finish tasks, and to dissect and solve problems. This is where reading, writing, and 'rithmetic create a masterly whole.

Globe and Lobe

The brain is not only divided into parts, it is also divided into two distinct hemispheres: the right and the left. The two work in tandem to make the whole "greater than its parts." The left hemisphere, for example, provides the ability to speak in most people. The right hemisphere gives that speech its lilt, color, and dialect. When a head injury occurs in the left hemisphere, the functions that are affected usually occur on the right side. Similarly, an accident in the right hemisphere will create problems in left-sided functions of the body.

Not only are there two hemispheres, but there are four "quarters" or lobes of the brain. Their functions are also at risk if a head injury occurs in their "section." These are the four "quarters":

➤ Frontal lobes are the most crucial part of the brain in terms of intellect, emotion, organizational and executive skills, and personality.

➤ Temporal lobes hold the bulk of the memory. They also make sense of "incoming information" and decide where it should go within the brain.

➤ Parietal lobes control the sense of touch, as well as the ability for reading comprehension and understanding spatial relationships.

➤ Occipital lobes are responsible for sight.

Knowing where a head injury occurred—in which part of the brain, which hemisphere, and which lobe—can help pinpoint the functions that will be affected.

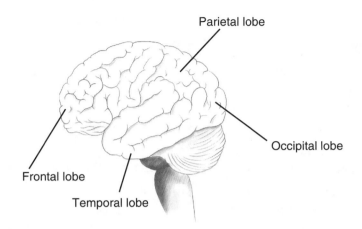

Parietal lobe

Occipital lobe

Frontal lobe

Temporal lobe

The brain is divided into four distinct lobes, which are responsible for very specific functions.

Working Together

Like all good corporations, the parts of the brain work in concert, ricocheting messages back and forth from nerve ends to the cerebrum, from the limbic system to the diencephalon, from the heart to the mind, from thoughts to feelings, from sensations to responses. The messages sent back and forth within the brain are propelled by a combination of electrical impulses and chemical conductors. This bustling network of electrochemical nerve fibers is made possible by three major allies: neurons, neurotransmitters, and synapses.

Neurons are simply brain cells. They nestle microscopically close together with liquidy spaces, called *synapses*, in between them. To pass electronically through one end of a neuron to the next, a message has to jump over the "impasse" that is the synapse. Neurons release chemicals called *neurotransmitters* at the synapse crossroad to help move the electrical impulses along (literally jumping the messages from one neuron cell to another). The type of chemical secreted, the amount released, and the pattern it creates is all encoded in the neurons. They sit in the brain fluid, silent and watchful like wallflowers, waiting for messages to come along so they can charge up their batteries. Basically, one specific neurotransmitter will be activated by an electrical impulse to carry the message to the next neuron waiting for its electric "hit."

All these goings-on, all these messages and responses, desires and actions, occur in less time than it takes to blink an eye! Scientists and physicians call it a precise machine. Poets call it a miracle. Whatever it is, the brain can (excuse the pun) boggle the mind.

> **First Aids**
> *Neurotransmitters* are the unique chemical messages released at the synapse. *Neurons* (nerve cells) make and store one or more of these messages, and some neurons even recapture the messengers and recycle them to be used again.

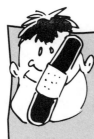

Before You Put the Band-Aid On

The skull might look smooth in Halloween costumes, but inside, there are ridges and bumps all over it. When someone falls down the stairs or hits her head on a steering wheel, the brain jiggles back and forth in its skull home.

Where does the injury usually begin? Right in front: right smack dab in the frontal lobe, where the intellectual, perceptual, and other higher-functioning skills lie.

The most dangerous damage from head injuries is often internal, where's it's invisible to the eye. If a person hits his head, say, on the side of a boat, the brain, which is floating in its cranial sac inside the skull, bangs back and forth and risks damage with each blow. When the brain hits against the inside wall of the skull, it starts to swell. It is this swelling that causes most symptoms of traumatic brain injury.

In addition to the bang-up job and the swelling, there's one more aspect to brain injury that can cause chaos. It's the jiggling of the brain, back and forth and from front to back, in an abrupt acceleration/deceleration movement. This makes the brain hit the skull ridges even more, causing rips, bruising, and hemorrhaging in the brain.

Bump? Concussion? Types of Brain Injury

Depending on the power of the "bang" and the location, a brain injury can be anything from a minor bump that goes away in a few days to a severe head injury that leaves the victim lying in a coma for a long time. Most head injuries are closed. This means that an observer can't see any blood, bumps, or bruises, but it doesn't mean that all those things aren't occurring inside the skull! You must rely on your powers of observation. Look for signs that are similar to any illness: nausea, chills, shock, dizziness, and disorientation.

A Bump Is a Lump

If a person merely bumps his or her head on, say, a cabinet door or a dresser drawer, chances are it will hurt, but the pain will subside soon. He might have a headache and even a lump where he bumped it, but he shouldn't notice any other symptoms. An ice compress and some aspirin should do the trick, especially when combined with a small nap (that stops movement for a while).

If the bump doesn't subside within 24 hours and/or if the person experiences nausea, chills, dizziness, or a spacey feeling that doesn't go away, he should call the doctor immediately.

A Blow to the Head: A Concussion

A *concussion* can be anything from a temporary loss of consciousness to that "ding" a baseball player hears in his head for 10 minutes after being socked by a hardball. The effects of a concussion can be additive or commutative, as it is in "punch-drunk" fighters, who eventually become unable to perform in the ring.

You should always seek medical help if a concussion is suspected. Your physician can determine if any neurological damage has been done, and he or she can begin rehabilitation treatment to prevent the damage from increasing.

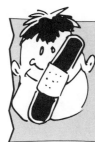

Before You Put the Band-Aid On

The brain seldom works alone. Many times, that twisting, pulling, bang-up job that takes place inside the skull also affects the nerve fibers in the neck—which connect to the spinal cord. The result can be a coma and/or paralysis.

Fractured Factions: A Skull Fracture

Of course, there are those terrible accidents that do puncture the skull. A bullet, a shard of glass, or a powerfully driven hard object can penetrate the skull and the brain, resulting in skull fracture and a brain injury. This open head injury puts a person further at risk because of the dangers of infection through the "open door." Treat a skull fracture as a medical emergency, not only because of the seriousness of the blow to the head, but also because of the risk of hemorrhaging and infection.

A Mild Head Injury: Five Good Signs

Although any head injury should be taken very seriously, 75 percent of all head injuries turn out to have mild consequences, which is good news. We suggest that you seek medical help for any suspected head injury, just to be certain that all is well and to prevent future problems (legal or medical). When a head injury is mild, the following five observations are usually true:

1. The injured person does not lose consciousness or is out only briefly. He or she may be confused for up to 20 minutes.

2. The person shows only mild physical symptoms of neurological damage including nausea, dizziness, or blurry vision (which can crop up anytime within three months of the accident).

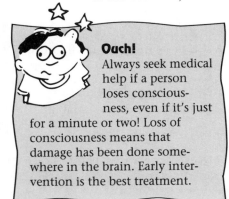

Ouch!
Always seek medical help if a person loses consciousness, even if it's just for a minute or two! Loss of consciousness means that damage has been done somewhere in the brain. Early intervention is the best treatment.

3. The person is treated in the emergency room and is not admitted at all, or he is hospitalized for no more than a week. He is ordered to rest and restrict his activities just long enough for the banged-up, bruised, jolted brain to heal and for the results of diagnostic tests to show little damage.

4. After three months, the injured person has few side effects.

5. There is no motor damage, and the injured person's "facilities" (his ability to think and solve problems) are intact.

Not Tonight. I Have a Headache.

One problem in pinpointing brain injury is the fact that symptoms and their accompanying neurological damage can crop up anytime within a year of the accident. Another problem is that some stubborn symptoms are there at the onset and just keep reoccurring and reoccurring.

These reoccurring and late-onset injuries are called post-concussive injuries. Some of the symptoms include recurring headaches, dizziness, and possible lapses in memory. Although many of these injuries are serious and real, they are becoming the newest fad for lawsuits. Like whiplash, these injuries are extremely difficult to prove or evaluate without repeated, detailed, and very expensive neuropsychiatric testing.

The best way to clear the air is to get an early evaluation from a doctor if a head injury is suspected—and always if a loss of consciousness occurs.

Treating a Mild Head Injury

Sometimes a head injury can start out minor and become serious a few hours later. If a person gets up and dusts himself off, but then goes home and goes to sleep, it could be a sign of a more serious condition. If you see that a person is sleeping excessively within 24 hours of a head injury, take him or her to the emergency ward.

It's always best to get medical help for any sort of head injury. If a person has blacked out, that help becomes imperative. Get an emergency team quickly. While you are waiting for help to arrive follow these steps:

1. Immobilize the victim as best you can, keeping him or her in a prone position because of possible spinal problems. (See Chapter 4 on vital emergencies.)

2. Avoid giving the victim alcohol, sedatives, or even water.

3. Observe the person for signs of shock and treat accordingly (see Chapter 3).

4. Keep the victim warm.

5. Use ice on the head to ease the pain while you wait.

6. If the victim is unconscious, time the length of the "blackout." This will help in determining a diagnosis later.

7. If the injured person is released under your care, watch him or her carefully for at least 48 hours. Make sure no symptoms recur. If they do, bring him or her back to the hospital as soon as possible.

Before You Put the Band-Aid On

It's vital that a person who has experienced a head injury participate in at least minimal rehabilitation exercises. Sometimes a head injury that appears to be mild at first glance can evolve into *post-concussion syndrome*, a condition that causes neurological capabilities and psychological emotions to slowly deteriorate over time. However, post-concussion syndrome can be stopped in its tracks with simple neurological and psychological rehabilitation techniques.

Danger Signs of a Serious Head Injury

Unfortunately, the other 25 percent of head injuries fall in the range between moderate damage and serious damage. If the injured person exhibits any of the characteristics listed here immediately after an accident, he or she probably has a moderate or serious injury.

Unconsciousness for 10 minutes or more

Seizures or convulsions

Inability to swallow or control elimination

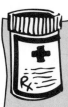

First Aids

A person is said to be in a coma if she is unconscious for more than 24 hours but her vital signs remain steady. Although the person appears to be sleeping, studies show that communication, touching, music, and even a recognized fragrance can help her come around.

Paralysis

Slurred words

Loss of memory; confusion that lasts for more than 15 minutes

Personality change, usually in aggressive, violent ways

Difficulty breathing

Pupils are unequal in size

If someone around you suffers what appears to be a moderate or serious head injury, first make sure that help is on the way (preferably from a trauma center), and then begin first aid. The next section covers the steps you should take to provide first aid for a serious or life-threatening head injury.

Emergency First Aid for Head Injuries

If you suspect serious head injury, you need to take care of three things right from the start:

Observe for signs of shock, a concussion, or a skull fracture.

Position the victim so he or she is immobile, in order to prevent further damage to both the brain and the spinal cord.

Treat scalp cuts and wounds for bleeding to avoid infection.

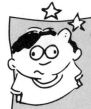

Ouch!

Do not give a person who has suffered a head injury any food or water. Both can induce vomiting—which can create breathing problems in a semiconscious or unconscious person. Note that ice packs won't help either. The best medicine is to get the person to a hospital—fast.

If you're in a situation where you need to provide help to a person who has experienced a severe head injury, take care to lend the following first aid:

1. Immediately call for help.

2. See if the injured person is unconscious. Note the length of time the unconsciousness lasts.

3. Look for bleeding from the eyes, nose, or ears. This doesn't have to be bright red blood; it can be something like brown discoloration around the rims of the eyes. This bleeding can be a sign of internal hemorrhaging. Keep the injured person in a prone position, face up.

4. If the injured person is conscious and does not appear to have a neck injury, place a pillow under his head and turn his face to the side.

5. While you are waiting for help, treat any scalp wounds. Clean cuts thoroughly, cover them with gauze, and apply tape that's firm but not constricting.

6. Look for outwardly physical signs of brain injury. These can include:

Severe headaches	Convulsions
Slurred words	Vomiting
Loss of vision or double vision	Loss of short-term memory
Bruising behind the ear or around the eyes	Clear or bloody fluid seeping from the ear, nose, or mouth
Unequal pupils	Weakness or paralysis in limbs

7. If any of the signs described in step 6 appears before an emergency medical team shows up, immobilize the injured person (see Chapter 4). This is crucial for preventing any more damage to the brain, spinal cord, or neck.

8. After the injured person has been released from medical care, he or she should be watched for the symptoms described in step 6 for at least 48 hours. If the symptoms recur, the victim should again seek emergency medical care as quickly as possible.

If the person you're helping has been knocked unconscious by the head injury, do not be surprised if she is in a highly agitated state when she becomes conscious. People who have been unconscious don't just open their eyes and yawn—contrary to what you see in Hollywood movies. They usually shake their heads and kick their feet, and they might pull at tubes that are hooked up to them. And, more than likely, they won't have a clue as to where they are or what happened—or even who you are sitting in the corner with tears in your eyes.

The longer a person is unconscious, the more agitated he or she may be upon recovery. Believe it or not, this is a characteristic you want to see. Agitation implies brain activity. Because the injured person is moving, shaking, and acting up, you know that she is alive and that the brain is functioning. Try to keep the person calm and still until medical help arrives. On the other hand, if the injured person doesn't move when she wakes up, or if her eyes stay focused in the distance, the head injury has probably caused damage to the brain.

The Least You Need to Know

➤ If you suspect a serious head injury, don't forget OPT: *Observe* the person for signs of a concussion, skull fracture, or shock. *Position* the person so that he or she is immobile. *Treat* any scalp cuts or bruises for bleeding.

➤ A bump on the head whose only symptom is pain does not usually require immediate medical care. But if the person begins to sleep excessively within the first 24 hours, or if the bump does not recede within a day or two, or if other physical symptoms of head injury occur, get the patient to a doctor!

➤ Signs of traumatic head injury include unconsciousness, loss of memory, blurred vision, paralysis, slurred speech, and severe headache. Always get emergency medical help fast for these head injuries!

➤ Internal bleeding in the head might not be visible by the naked eye, but there are clues. If fluids seep out of the mouth, ears, or nose, or if the victim fails to improve or actually seems to get worse, there might be some hemorrhaging inside.

➤ Note the length of time the injured person is unconscious. It can be a factor in the later success of rehabilitation.

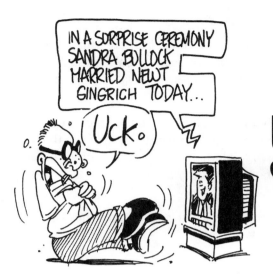

Heart Attacks and Strokes

Heart attacks are not something we like to think about—until we're older anyway. The same goes for strokes. These are problems that happen to other people, in other lives. Unfortunately, statistics show that people are having heart attacks at increasingly younger ages.

Coronary heart disease is the leading cause of death in this country, and strokes come in as the third leading cause of death. We're not asking you to dwell on these conditions. But, like animal bites or bumps on the head, they can happen to you or someone around you—when you least expect it.

If you know something about these killers, you can put your first aid expertise to use and perhaps save a life! This chapter explains how.

What Leads Up to a Heart Attack?

Although heart attacks often seem to come from out of the blue, they are usually the result of years of "abuse." Cigarette smoking, high blood pressure, high cholesterol, obesity, family medical history, diabetes, and a sedentary lifestyle are all factors that can contribute to an eventual heart attack.

Ironically, except for a family history of heart conditions and genetic programming, the risk factors for heart attacks are within your control. Losing weight, eating foods that are low in fat and high in fiber, exercising, taking high blood pressure medication (if necessary), and quitting smoking can all ensure not only a healthy lifestyle, but a healthy heart.

However, starting and maintaining a healthier lifestyle is easier said than done. And often, despite our best intentions, things go awry.

Warning Signs of a Heart Attack

Heart attacks can really be divided into two separate conditions: angina and myocardial infarction.

Angina is temporary pain that can be caused a spasm in the heart's coronary arteries. It is usually the result of an inadequate blood flow to the heart caused by overexertion of the heart combined with a build-up of cholesterol. Rest and/or nitroglycerin pills placed under the tongue can get halt pain from angina within five minutes. Most people who are prone to angina carry nitroglycerin pills with them at all times. Angina usually occurs during exertion or exercise. If it occurs when a person is at rest, it could be a sign of a possible heart attack. The person should seek medical help immediately.

Myocardial infarction (MI) and *cardiovascular disease (CVS)* are other names for a heart attack. Here, a piece of the heart muscle is actually destroyed when a coronary artery becomes closed and completely "shuts down." Heart attacks do not occur only during periods of overexertion (while shoveling snow, for example); these serious heart attacks might occur several hours *after* a strenuous situation, exercise, or heavy meal, while a person is at rest. In fact, many heart attacks occur early in the morning (around 6:00 am), when the body is gearing up to start the day. If pain wakes you up in the morning, it's a serious warning sign of a possible heart attack. Seek medical help immediately!

The terrible, crushing pressure of heart pain occurs because blood and its life-giving oxygen cannot reach the heart muscle because of a clogged artery. The following symptoms can indicate a heart attack. If a person near you has *any* of these symptoms call for help and begin first aid measures immediately.

➤ Uncomfortable pressure, fullness, squeezing, or pain in the center of the chest that lasts for more than two minutes.

➤ Pain that spreads out to the shoulders, neck, jaw, arms, and stomach.

➤ Gasping or shortness of breath that gets worse when lying flat.

➤ "Heartburn" pain that doesn't improve with antacids.

> **First Things First**
> It's difficult to exactly describe pressure or pain in the chest. Some people describe it as a "tightness" or a "crushing feeling" or like a "herd of elephants trampling over my heart."

➤ Chest pain combined with lightheadedness, severe anxiety, heavy sweating, pale skin and bluish lips, irregular or rapid pulse, or nausea.

Chest pain doesn't always mean a heart attack. In fact, most chest pains aren't heart attacks at all, but are merely symptoms of indigestion, muscle strain, shingles, or respiratory ailments. However, if any of the "red flags" appear, it's better to be embarrassed in the emergency room than to be...well, dead.

If You Think Someone Is Having a Heart Attack...

Although a heart attack is a frightening proposition, there is good news. With today's sophisticated equipment, procedures, and diagnostic tools for treating heart attacks, people who suffer an attack can go on to live long, productive lives. But there is an operative word: help. Getting help fast is the only way to possibly prevent disaster. Even if you're sure that the stab of pain you feel is indigestion, go to the doctor. Better to be safe than sorry.

> **Ouch!**
> Never attempt to drive a person who is having a heart attack to the hospital yourself. The cramped conditions of a car will make it difficult for you to perform CPR, check vital signs, or even keep the ill person comfortable. Only an ambulance is equipped to deal with heart conditions, unexpected emergencies, and the heavy flow of traffic.

1. Immediately call 911 for help.

2. If you know CPR (cardio-pulmonary resuscitation), begin it immediately if necessary. See the information on CPR at the end of this chapter and in Chapter 3 for details.

3. If you don't know CPR, sit the person up or have him or her rest in a semi-reclining position, whichever is more comfortable.

4. Loosen any clothing around the neck that's restrictive, such as a collar, necktie, shirt, or scarf.

5. Observe and watch the ABCs you learned about in Chapter 1. Make sure the Airways are open, that Breathing is regular, and that Circulation is steady. If the ill person loses consciousness, continue to check his or her pulse. If he or she vomits, turn the head to the side and clean the mouth.

6. If the ill person has angina medication, place it under his or her tongue. If the pain goes away, chances are the person has had an angina attack and will soon be fine (although a visit to the emergency room is still a good idea to remove all doubt). Do not give nitroglycerin pills unless a doctor has prescribed them for that person!

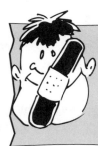

Before You Put the Band-Aid On

Like nicotine withdrawal medication and seasickness medication, nitroglycerin now comes in patches. Patches can keep angina attacks at bay anywhere from 12–24 hours. Check with your physician about this new medication if you or someone you love has been diagnosed with angina.

The Difference Between Strokes and Heart Attacks

The National Stroke Association defines a stroke as "a sudden disruption of the blood supply to a part of the brain, which, in turn, disrupts the body function controlled by that brain area." In short, you might call a stroke a "heart attack" that occurs in the brain.

There are technically four different types of strokes, but all of them have the same basic description: a blood clot or clogged artery prevents blood from continuing through the brain. The areas on the other side of this "medical dam" cannot receive the nutrient-rich blood they need to function. The result? Like a lawn that isn't watered in the heat of summer, the brain cells dry up and die.

The "Laps" a Stroke Swims

This is what happens when someone experiences a stroke. An artery wall in the brain or neck becomes clogged, and blood can't get past the clog. As a result, the brain cells beyond the clog literally die from the lack of oxygen-rich blood. When those cells die, the person loses whatever function those brain cells controlled.

Because we know that certain areas of the brain control certain functions, we can predict the effects of a stroke based on the location of the blockage. If the blockage occurs near the front of the brain, it can affect such things as organization skills, memory, communication, and problem solving. If it occurs lower down, near the brainstem, it can cause unconsciousness and an inability to breathe, swallow, or control elimination.

In addition, which side (hemisphere) of the brain the stroke occurs on determines its side effects and which body functions are affected. (See Chapter 16 for a full explanation of the right and left hemispheres of the brain.) If the blockage occurs anywhere on the right side of the brain, it can result in the following conditions:

➤ Paralysis or weakness on the left side of the body

➤ Disorientation

➤ Extreme emotional highs and lows

➤ Excessive talking

➤ An inability to perform routine tasks such as brushing the teeth or buttoning a shirt

First Aids
If the stroke happens in the brain itself, it is called *thrombosis*. If a blood clot in another part of the body (either the neck or the heart) breaks away from that artery wall and travels up to the brain, the stroke that occurs is called *embolic*.

If the stroke occurs anywhere on the left side of the brain, it can produce the following results:

➤ Paralysis or weakness on the right side of the body

➤ Depression

➤ An inability to understand language

➤ Trouble speaking

➤ Memory problems

➤ Decreased attention span

First Aids
The right and left sides of the brain are referred to as *hemispheres*. The right side controls more of a person's emotions, creativity, and abstract thinking. The left hemisphere controls more of the language skills, logic, perception, and organization.

Although a stroke, or an *infarction* as it is officially called, can occur in younger people, it is usually the result of the build-up over the years that clogs, narrows, and decreases the resilience of arteries leading to the brain.

Like heart attacks, the risk factors that may lead to stroke include such unhealthy lifestyle choices as cigarette smoking, obesity, and uncontrolled high blood pressure, combined with factors that we can't do anything about, such as family medical history, individual medical history, and diabetes.

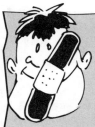

Before You Put the Band-Aid On

A Transient Ischemic Attack, or TIA, is a true warning sign of a full-fledged stroke. A mini-stroke that lasts no more than 24 hours, a TIA could be compared to tremors that occur before an earthquake. Heed nature's warning. You can make changes in your lifestyle, take certain medication, and (in very serious cases) have an operation to ensure that you won't suffer a full-fledged stroke.

Warning Signs of a Stroke or TIA (Transient Ischemic Attack)

A stroke can occur as suddenly as a heart attack—when a person is walking down the street, driving a car, or sitting in a rowboat in the middle of a lake. With a stroke, however, the brain doesn't just shut down all at once. Depending on the location of the blockage, there may be any of several warning signs. (As realtors always say, "Location is everything.")

With a TIA, the following symptoms last no more than 24 hours. More often than not, however, they signal the onset of a stroke:

➤ Sudden weakness or numbness of the face, arm, or leg on one side of the body only

➤ Sudden loss of speech, or trouble finding the right words

➤ Inability to comprehend what is being said

➤ Sudden dimness of vision bilateral (both eyes) or loss of vision in one eye

➤ A sudden, very severe headache

➤ A sudden episode of dizziness or unsteadiness, or even a sudden fall

➤ Loss of bladder or bowel control

➤ Unconsciousness

➤ Very flushed face

Providing Emergency Treatment for a Stroke Until Help Arrives

As we've said over and over again, try to stay calm! Follow these first aid basics until an emergency medical team arrives on the scene.

1. Call for help.

2. Put the ill person in a semi-reclining position, if possible.

3. Loosen clothing around the neck and chest.

4. Check the victim's airways for blockage. Begin mouth-to-mouth resuscitation, if necessary (see Chapter 3).

5. Dab cool washcloths or cold compresses on the patient's neck and face.

6. If the person vomits, turn his head to the side and clean all vomit from his mouth.

7. Treat for shock, especially if the person is unconscious (see Chapter 3).

8. If the ill person has a muscle spasm or a seizure, follow first aid procedures for seizures and convulsions (as covered in Chapter 25).

The First Two Hours: A Window of Opportunity

The first two hours after a heart attack or a stroke are the most crucial. Any damage done by a stroke can be contained if you can get the ill person to a trauma center or emergency room as fast as possible. If administered during this two-hour "window," the proper medication can not only stop stroke damage, it can even revive the seemingly dead brain cells that have already caused malfunction. Studies show that the sooner a person begins rehabilitation after a stroke, the greater his or her chances are for a moderate to excellent recovery. And if it is a TIA and the person recovers on his or her own, medication and/or surgery can prevent a stroke in the future.

When a person has a heart attack, those first two hours can literally mean the difference between life and death. If the heart stops beating anytime during those two hours, it causes sudden death. Even if help arrives soon after the onset of a heart attack, if the heart has stopped beating, the caregivers have only a few minutes to reverse the damage. Without the heart pumping blood, the brain cannot get the needed oxygen-rich blood. Therefore, brain damage is a distinct possibility.

But there is real hope—and help. Its initials are CPR.

Do You Know CPR?

CPR is short for cardio-pulmonary resuscitation. If this procedure is begun immediately after someone has a heart attack, it can save his life. When performed properly, CPR can keep the blood circulating until help arrives. At that point, trained medical staff can use more sophisticated treatment en route to the hospital.

Although similar to mouth-to-mouth resuscitation, CPR is much more precise, involving step-by-step movements with the hands, mouth, and arms that must be concisely and rhythmically performed continuously until help arrives. In fact, CPR cannot be interrupted for any more than *fifteen* seconds once it's started!

CPR is not difficult, but you need to be trained to do it so that you can do it without thinking. You can learn this skill in one or two sessions with a trained instructor. Almost every hospital offers CPR classes during the year, including special sessions on CPR for children. You can also take CPR classes at your local YMCA.

Although CPR classes do cost some money, it is not exorbitant. (There is, after all, no price tag on life.) During the month of February—which has been dubbed "Heart Healthy Month"—many hospitals offer specials on CPR, sometimes giving classes for free or for as little as $5.00. Check with your local hospital or YMCA for information about CPR classes.

For more information on heart disease and its effects, prevention, and treatment, contact your local chapter of the American Heart Association (in the white pages of your phone book). Or you can simply call or write the American Heart Association at its national center:

American Heart Association National Center
7272 Greenville Avenue
Dallas, Texas
1-800-AHA-USA-1
(1-800-242-8721)
Web site: http://www.amhrt.org

The Least You Need to Know

➤ A stroke or heart attack does not have to be catastrophic. You can help while you wait for assistance.

➤ Symptoms of a heart attack include a feeling of great pressure on the heart muscle, a shot of pain down the left arm and shoulder, shortness of breath that doesn't ease up, and building anxiety.

➤ The first two hours after a stroke or a heart attack are the most crucial.

➤ Angina is a pain in the heart that is usually caused by a combination of cholesterol build-up and exertion. Nitroglycerin tablets can immediately ease the pain.

➤ Never feel foolish seeking help when there's a possibility of a heart attack. If you have a case of indigestion and antacids don't seem to do the trick, go to the emergency ward. It's better to be safe than sorry!

➤ If you know CPR, immediately begin the procedure if there is no pulse. If a person is not breathing, perform mouth-to-mouth resuscitation.

➤ A stroke can have various symptoms, depending on the area of the brain where it occurs.

➤ A TIA is a "warning" stroke. Its symptoms include a sudden numbness of the body, sudden loss of speech, sudden dimness of vision, severe headache, abrupt dizziness, loss of bladder control, unconsciousness, and a very flushed face, but those symptoms pass within 24 hours.

➤ The risk of both strokes and heart attacks are affected by a person's lifestyle. Eating right, exercising, taking high blood pressure medicine regularly (if necessary), refraining from smoking, and losing weight will all decrease a person's chances.

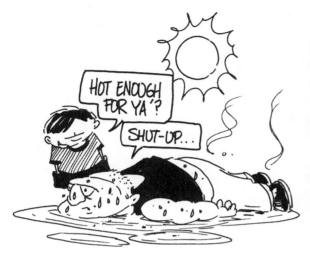

Chapter 18

Heat Prostration, Sunstroke, Hypothermia, and Frostbite

In This Chapter

➤ What exactly is heat prostration?

➤ Symptoms of sun and heat overexposure

➤ First aid measures to cool the body down before medical help arrives

➤ Knowing and treating frostbite

➤ Symptoms of hypothermia (overexposure to cold)

Once upon a time, people gleefully left for vacation with suntan oils and sun reflectors in hand, anticipating spending hours and hours in the sun and getting a great tan. Today, however, we know that too much sun is harmful. Medical experts suggest that we build up a tan slowly (if we must have one), stay out of the sun during the hours of direct sunlight (11:00–2:00), and never even walk out the door of the house without a hat or some sunblock.

The fact is that not only can too much sun age us, but it can cause skin cancer—specifically deadly melanoma that can kill if it's not caught in time. But skin damage occurs over time, over years in fact.

On a daily basis, there are other sun-related conditions that can present sudden problems, and those problems need first aid care. This chapter describes heat prostration (also called heat exhaustion) and its partner in crime, sunstroke, and arms you with the first aid steps to deal with them.

You'll also find information about a different extreme: winter cold. Hypothermia can be just as deadly as heat prostration. It is especially common among the elderly, outdoor hikers, and people who do not have adequate heat. Frostbite occurs as a result of extreme overexposure to cold. It can accompany hypothermia, or it can be a first aid emergency all by itself.

But first, the sun…

When the Sun Heats Up

Sun and heat-related illnesses usually occur under one or more of the following conditions:

> ➤ In the early summer when people have not yet adapted themselves to the hot weather usually associated with the "dog days" of July and August.

> ➤ During excessive exercising in the hot sun (running, bicycling, or doing push-ups during Army drill).

> ➤ While in the midst of an unexpected "heat wave."

People use the words heat prostration, heat exhaustion, and sunstroke interchangeably. In reality, *heat prostration* and *heat exhaustion* are the same: a condition that occurs in an "overheated" body. Like an overheated car, the body's cooling mechanisms just can't keep up, and a person begins to feel as if he has the flu. He might be confused; he might feel chilled; his skin might be clammy to the touch; his face might become flushed. Heat prostration (or exhaustion) is rarely life-threatening, but it must be treated. If you don't take care of an over-heated body, unconsciousness, shock, and even death, can result.

Sunstroke has symptoms similar to heat prostration, with one major difference: the body's cooling mechanism has completely stopped. It's not running slowly, it's stalled. Obviously, this element makes sunstroke and its consequent treatment more serious. It's important to recognize the subtle differences between heat prostration and sunstroke. Let's go over each one now, covering everything from symptoms to first aid care.

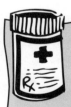

First Aids

A "heat wave" is more than a temperature over 90 degrees. For meteorologists to officially call it a heat wave, the high temperature must be combined with high humidity and a lack of wind. In other words, the air is close, hot, and stuffy… so you feel like you're trapped under a heavy wool blanket.

Symptoms of Heat Prostration (Exhaustion)

If you notice someone suddenly experiencing any of the following symptoms, you can bet that heat prostration (or exhaustion) has made an unwelcome visit.

Sudden high temperature (but less than 104 degrees)

Hot and flushed skin that might be clammy to the touch

Muscle or stomach cramps

Nausea and/or vomiting

Headache

Profuse sweating

Rapid pulse

Dizziness

Treating Heat Prostration or Exhaustion

Heat exhaustion is not usually a life-threatening condition. The two important rules to remember regarding heat prostration and exhaustion are:

1. Get the ill person out of the sun.

2. Replace the body's lost fluids and salt by having the person drink lots of water, Gatorade, decaffeinated iced tea, or juice.

3. Cool the person's body with fans, cool towels, or sprays.

4. Keep the sufferer out of the sun for the next 12–24 hours.

A person who has suffered a bout of heat prostration needs to rest. Like that overheated car, he or she needs to cool off before "revving" up the engine again. The best bet is a full day of rest (at least 12 hours) during which time he or she should catch up on lost fluids and give the body time to repair its systems. Once a person suffers heat prostration, he is more vulnerable to another occurrence of it (and to the more serious sunstroke). So relax and enjoy your time off!

> **Ouch!**
> When suffering from heat exhaustion, you might be tempted to jump into the pool or the lake to cool off. Don't do it! If you go into the water with a case of heat exhaustion, you could end up with cramps. Worse, you could pass out or have a seizure, which might lead to drowning.

Symptoms of Sunstroke

Sunstroke (or heat stroke) is much more serious than heat prostration. You might call sunstroke the "evil cousin" that comes to visit when heat exhaustion is not treated promptly. In fact, because the body's cooling mechanisms shut down, sunstroke can be life-threatening. Its symptoms include:

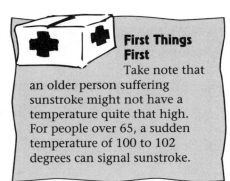

First Things First

Take note that an older person suffering sunstroke might not have a temperature quite that high. For people over 65, a sudden temperature of 100 to 102 degrees can signal sunstroke.

Sudden, extremely high temperature (104 degrees and higher)

Hot, flushed, and very dry skin

A total absence of sweating

Rapid pulse

Confusion

Unconsciousness

Convulsions

Treating Sunstroke, Step-by-Cooling-Step

It's hard enough to put suntan lotion on a person when it's hot, sticky, and humid outside and the sun is beating down unmercifully. Treating a person who has fallen victim to these weather conditions is doubly difficult. But, despite the heat, you must keep a cool head and follow these steps.

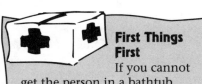

First Things First

If you cannot get the person in a bathtub, wrap him in water-soaked, cool sheets and use a fan or the cool setting on a hair dryer to blow air on his body. You can also give the person a sponge bath with cool water from a pitcher or bucket. (But make sure the water is not *too* cold; comfort combined with effectiveness is the key.)

1. Immediately call for help. Sunstroke is a life-threatening emergency.

2. Immerse the ill person in a half-filled tub of cool water in an attempt to lower body temperature as quickly as possible.

3. Sponge bathe the ill person with cool water.

4. Once you get the temperature down, briskly towel the person dry.

5. If the patient is conscious and coherent, you can offer him plain water while he is waiting for medical attention, but do not give him caffeinated drinks such as coffee, tea, or soda.

6. Once you've taken these emergency measures, make sure the victim gets medical attention—even if the person appears to have made a full recovery.

A Cautionary Note: It's Not Nice to Make Fun of Mother Nature

The sun can be a relaxing friend or a life-threatening enemy. Under any extreme weather conditions, you should do things in moderation. When the weather's cold, you don't go outside without a heavy coat, hat, gloves, and boots. When you get too cold, you stop ice-skating and sip some hot chocolate.

The sun also requires your respect. Sitting in the sun is fine if you replenish yourself with liquids, keep the length of time short, and wear plenty of sunblock. Getting too much exercise or exposure in hot, seething, humid weather is as irresponsible as wearing a T-shirt outside in below zero weather. Heed these tips to avoid the devastating effects of sun and heat:

➤ Restrict tennis and running activities to early morning or evening hours, when the weather is cooler and the sun less intense.

➤ Carry a container of water with you at all times.

➤ Drink at least eight glasses of water a day.

➤ Wear cool clothing, such as cottons and synthetics that "lick up" sweat and keep you cool.

➤ Always wear sunscreen and a visor or cotton cap when you're outside.

➤ Don't look directly at the sun, and wear good protective sunglasses to avoid eye damage.

The Other Extreme: Hypothermia

The fact is that extreme temperatures can spell problems unless you take proper precautions. Just as too much heat and sun can cause illness, so can extreme cold.

Hypothermia is the condition that results from a drastic loss of body heat as a result of overexposure of the cold. A person suffering from hypothermia will have a sudden, abnormally low body temperature (below 95 degrees) which, in turn, will slow down important physiological activity such as like breathing, swallowing, and circulation of blood.

Those most at risk for hypothermia include the elderly, outdoor hikers, mountain climbers (like the unfortunate sportspeople who attempted to climb Mount Everest), and those who are accidentally exposed to cold from car accidents, ice accidents, sudden winter storms and winds, faulty heating systems, and poorly insulated outerwear.

The symptoms of hypothermia occur suddenly and abruptly. They include:

Fatigue

Depressed, slow pulse

Low blood pressure

A tremendous "need" to sleep

Weakness

Slow, barely noticeable breathing

Drowsiness

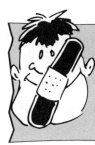

Before You Put the Band-Aid On

Sometimes hypothermia is a good thing. Hypothermia is actually induced deliberately to decrease metabolism during certain surgeries and in organs due for transplantation.

Hypothermia is rarely life-threatening—if it is treated quickly enough! Unfortunately, many people die from it, especially elderly men and women who live alone in poorly maintained apartments or houses. If you need to administer first aid for hypothermia, follow these steps:

1. Get the person indoors to warmth, but avoid radiators and fireplaces. These offer too extreme a change and can cause more harm.

2. Cover the person with a loose, warm blanket to prevent further loss of body heat. Getting under the cover with them provides natural heat from your body, which will also help warm up the victim.

3. If the person is conscious, appears lucid, and can swallow, you can offer him or her something warm and soothing to sip—but avoid alcohol.

4. If possible, observe the person for several hours. Cardiac arrest is not uncommon during hypothermia, and you'll need to be nearby to administer first aid, if necessary! (See Chapter 17 for details on heart attacks.)

The Nip of Winter: Frostbite

Frostbite is the cold kissing cousin of hypothermia. It's quite common and almost never life-threatening (although it can be serious enough for a person to lose part of a limb!). It "loves" cold winter weather, especially when low temperatures are combined with a cold wind or wet conditions.

Some body parts are more susceptible to frostbite than others. As you might guess, the extremities are most at risk because they are more exposed to extreme weather conditions. By extremities, we mean the nose, ears, fingers, toes, and chin. You don't wear that ski mask, thick heavy socks, and insulated mittens for nothing! You'll know you are suffering from frostbite when the affected body part starts to tingle or ache slightly, and eventually becomes numb.

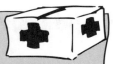

First Things First

You can recognize frostbite by its color. Frostbitten fingers or toes will first be bright red. Then they'll turn gray, and then stark, icy white. (Darker skin will ultimately become an ashy gray color.)

Frostbite first aid treatment is easy to follow. As soon as you recognize its telltale symptoms, immediately begin this treatment procedure. If you get help quickly, loss of limbs can be avoided!

1. Call for medical help immediately.

2. Get the person in from the cold as quickly as possible and remove any wet or icy clothing.

3. Protect the frozen area of the body, "thawing" it out with lukewarm water. If water isn't available, use a warm, woolen blanket or natural body heat. (For example, you could put frostbitten fingers into the armpits—if you could stand it.) Do *not* use a hair dryer, as it is too hot.

4. Within half an hour, feeling will return—and with it will come a lot of pain. The area will also become red and swollen. Although this might seem horrible, it is a good thing. It's a sign that blood is beginning to circulate in the area again.

5. Once the body part is thawed, keep it warm, dry, and clean until you see a physician.

6. If blisters appear, apply an antibacterial ointment and a loose, sterile dressing.

Before You Put the Band-Aid On

You might be tempted to massage the body part in question, thinking you'll warm it with your touch. Don't do that. Massage can cause tissue damage to frostbitten areas. And, as a matter of fact, if there's a chance that the ear or toe or whatever will refreeze before help arrives on the scene, don't even attempt to thaw. Thawing and refreezing is worse for your body than leaving the frostbite alone for the moment!

The Least You Need to Know

➤ Heat prostration is less serious than sunstroke, but it does require some first aid.

➤ Recognize the main differences between heat prostration and sunstroke: With heat prostration, the victim has a temperature less than 104 degrees and sweats profusely. With sunstroke, the temperature is higher than 104 degrees, and there is an absence of sweat. (In the elderly, this temperature will be lower, from 100 to 102 degrees.)

➤ When someone suffers from heat prostration or sunstroke, get him out of the sun, try to lower the body temperature (bathing in cool water helps), and provide noncaffeinated liquids.

➤ Sunstroke is a life-threatening emergency. Always call for help!

➤ Avoid hypothermia by wearing ski masks, insulated mittens, and warm, heavy socks when you must be outdoors in cold weather.

➤ Hypothermia results in a rapid drop in body temperature. Get a person suffering from this condition into a warm area as quickly as possible. Cover him or her with a blanket. Watch for any possible sign of cardiac arrest.

➤ Frostbite is a condition in which the tissue literally becomes frozen. Treat by "thawing" the body part with lukewarm water. Do not use massage.

➤ After 30 minutes, an area that has been affected by frostbite will begin to hurt; it will turn red and swell. Don't be alarmed. It means that blood is circulating in the area once again.

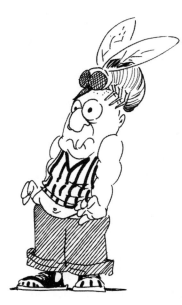

Chapter 19

Insect Bites—from Bee Stings to Ticks—and Other Skin Irritations

In This Chapter

➤ Treating bee stings without injuring yourself

➤ Ticks and signs of Lyme disease

➤ Step-by-step first aid for skin problems

➤ Knowing which spiders are poisonous and which are not

➤ What to do when the scorpion stings

➤ The ants that should not be let out of the "farm"

Ah, the pleasures of picnicking by a lake, or hiking through the desert, or relaxing under a tree in the woods and letting the breeze kiss your cheek. True, there's nothing like nature to soothe the nerves, calm the spirit, and rejuvenate the body. But like the scouts always say, "Be prepared."

A picnic can be ruined by a swarm of bees or several hundred bustling ants. A hike in the Southwest can bring you face-to-face with a scorpion. And the woods can be inhabited by critters carrying ticks. As if the pain of the bite isn't enough, you might get a dose of Lyme disease from an infected tick, or you might find that you're allergic to an insect bite when you exhibit a huge, red hive as a result. These situations don't have to spoil your fun. Simply turn to the appropriate pages in this chapter, and you'll find everything you need to administer first aid.

Bees and Wasps

When a bee or wasp stings you, the distinctions that make one insect a bee and one a wasp hardly matter. However, it's important for you to know one distinguishing factor: wasps are more aggressive than bees.

Bees are "vegetarian," feeding their young only nectar, and they live in hives built from natural wax secretions. Bumblebees and honeybees simply look for nectar and pollen to take back to their hives for food. If you leave them alone, chances are, they will ignore your un-honeyed arm or leg.

Wasps (also called hornets) are more belligerent. They, too, go after pollen and nectar, but because their tongues are shorter, they are unable to get nectar from many flowers that bees can. Therefore, wasps feed their young other insects in addition to nectar. Wasps build their nests from paper or wood, or they burrow into the ground. Yellow jackets are a type of wasp.

A honeybee (left) looks similar to a yellow jacket (right), but it is much less aggressive.

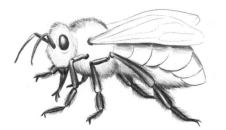 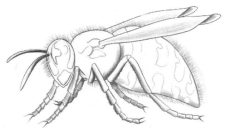

At First Bite: Symptoms of Bee and Wasp Stings

One sting from a bee or a wasp will cause a burning feeling at the site of the bite. It will hurt—probably a lot—but the pain will be localized. The site might swell, turn red, and itch. Multiple stings are more serious. They can cause fever, headache, muscle cramps, and drowsiness.

Stings are not usually life-threatening, but they can be if you have an allergy to the bee's venom. Signs of allergic reaction include nausea, excessive swelling, trouble breathing, bluish face and lips, choking, shock, and unconsciousness. If someone is sensitive to bee stings or if someone receives multiple stings (which can create an allergic reaction even in non-allergic persons), call for emergency help immediately. Watch the victim's vital signs and treat for shock or breathing difficulties if necessary (see Chapter 3).

A Taste of Treatment

Another crucial difference between bees and wasps lies in what happens when they sting. When a bee stings, it leaves both its stinger and a venom sac inside the victim's skin. Even though there's retribution in the fact that the bee "committed suicide," its venom sac gets implanted in the skin and continues to release foreign secretions.

When a wasp stings, it leaves behind only a stinger, no excess venom. And sometimes it doesn't even leave the stinger. Sometimes the stinger stays intact on the insect, enabling it to sting again and again. It's not uncommon for one yellow jacket to sting seven or more times before its stinger "drops off" in a person's skin.

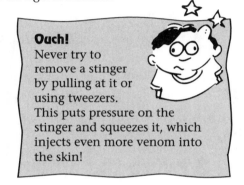

Ouch!
Never try to remove a stinger by pulling at it or using tweezers. This puts pressure on the stinger and squeezes it, which injects even more venom into the skin!

However, treatment is the same for bee stings (which leave venom sacs and stingers) and wasp stings (which leave stingers but no sacs).

1. If the stinger is clearly visible in the skin, gently "scoop" it out with the edge of a toothpick, a long fingernail, or a pocket knife.

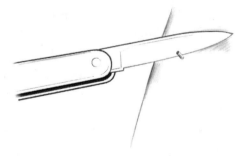

"Scoop" out the stinger with a knife, using an upward prying motion.

2. Wash the affected area with soap and cold water. Then apply ice in a compress or wrapped in a towel or cloth to alleviate pain and slow down the body's venom absorption. (Always wrap the ice before placing it on the skin; plain ice sticks and causes more irritation.)

3. Apply calamine lotion or a mixture of baking soda and water.

4. If the victim is not allergic, you can give him or her aspirin, ibuprofen, or acetaminophen to help relieve the pain. If that seems to take care of it, the treatment is finished. If you are treating a more serious bee sting or multiple stings, proceed with the steps.

5. For multiple stings, soak the entire affected area in cool water. If necessary, place the victim in a tub of cool water. Add one tablespoon of baking soda for every quart of water.

6. If the victim has an allergic reaction, call for emergency help. Then have the victim lie in a prone position. Keep the affected area immobile and, if possible, lower than the heart. This will slow down the venom's circulation.

7. Tie a strip of cloth, a belt, a watchband, or the sleeve of a shirt two to four inches above the affected area. The bandage should be snug, but loose enough to fit a finger underneath it. (This ensures that you are not completely cutting off circulation.)

8. If the affected area starts to swell near the strip of cloth, tie another strip two to four inches above the first. Then remove the first strip.

Beware the Spider

Spiders: Those creepy, crawly critters that have been the stuff of nightmares, horror movies, Halloween decorations, and cries that would wake the dead, "Kill it. Please. Eeeech!" Unfortunately, these arachnids (which is the scientific term for all sorts of spiders) get a bad rap. True, there a few types that are poisonous to man and should be avoided at all costs. But the garden-variety spider is usually harmless—and they even serve a good purpose on earth.

Spiders eat other insects, those pests that would eat your tomato plants and flowers. In the house, they'll eat pests you'd rather not have around. And if their webs aren't in clear sight, you're better off keeping the status quo.

Of course, there are spiders that bite—and some whose bite is poisonous. These bites require first aid treatment and medical care.

First Things First

It's not something you'd want to contemplate for a long period of time, but most garden-variety spiders *do* bite. Luckily, their tiny fangs are too short and their venom is too weak to inflict humans with much more injury than an itch.

A Guide to Common Spiders

To help you differentiate between the bad guys and the good guys, here's a brief description of the spiders you might see in your backyard or in your kitchen, depending on where in the United States you live.

Good Guys

Daddy longlegs are so called because of their thin, long legs; they are the "daddy" of long-legged spiders. Although they look creepy, they are absolutely harmless. They are uninterested in us *homo sapiens*. Instead, they usually stay outside, crawling on tree trunks, dancing through the grass, and moving across soil.

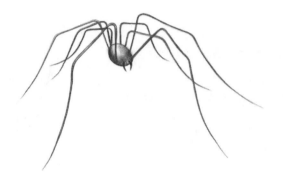

A daddy longlegs spider.

Common gray and gray/brown spiders are the ones you'll most likely find in your house. They're the ones who make those annoying webs on lampshades, fixtures, and bookshelves. Like all spiders, they have eight legs. Their legs are usually short, and their bodies are round. Like ordinary folks, these are ordinary spiders. They'll help you get rid of bugs better than flypaper.

Bad Guys

There are only three types of spiders to worry about. Their bites can hurt and definitely require first aid treatment.

Black widow spiders are the Queens of mean. You can recognize a black widow by the red or yellow hourglass marking on the underside of its belly. Only the female of the species is poisonous; she even kills the males after she has "used them" to get pregnant. Despite the wallop they pack, black widow spiders are quite small, measuring only about 3/4 inch in diameter. They are most commonly found in the Southwest.

Symptoms of a black widow's bite may include an immediate sharp, severe pain; immediate redness at the site; profuse sweating; nausea and stomach cramps; difficulty breathing; and a tingling, burning feeling throughout the body.

173

A black widow spider.

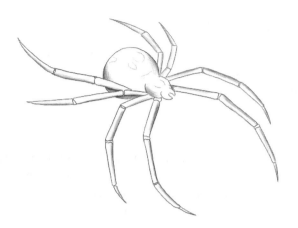

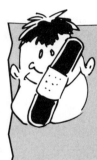

Before You Put the Band-Aid On

The myth that a black widow's bite might be fatal has been put to rest by many studies. Apparently, black widow spider bites cause a great deal of discomfort, but when the venom goes through your system, it does not leave "residue poison." Many people who have even been bitten twice live to tell the tale.

Violin or brown recluse spiders almost look like "strings" attached to small body. They are either yellow or tan and have a dark brown fiddle-like design on their backs. They are quite small, measuring only 1/2 to 5/8 of an inch in size.

A brown recluse (violin) spider.

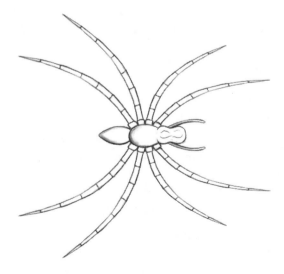

Symptoms of brown recluse spider bites include severe pain that occurs approximately eight hours after the bite; swelling at the bite site; blistering; chills and fever; aches and pains in the joints; nausea; and vomiting. There's a visual aid as well. Sometimes you can see an enlargement around the bite "target." It might have a dusky or dark center and red, raised, expanding edge.

Tarantulas really get a bad rap from humans. These large, fuzzy spiders might look like a reject from a horror movie, but in reality, they're not so bad. There are even people who (gulp!) keep them as pets. Although a tarantula's bite hurts, it's rarely fatal. And the bite itself usually causes nothing more than short-lived localized pain at the site. You'll most likely find tarantulas in shipments of bananas and other fruits from South America (and in James Bond movies).

Tarantula bites usually cause only short-term pain at the bite site; occasionally, though, they cause very intense pain at the site. Other possible symptoms include redness, swelling, a blistering and festered wound, numbness, difficulty breathing, nausea, and stomach cramps.

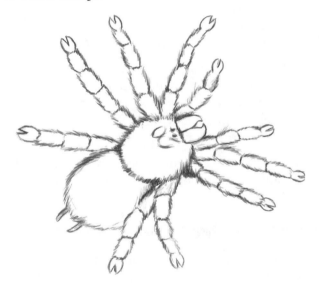

A tarantula.

Treating Spider Bites

The treatment for spider bites is the same whether a person is bitten by a black widow, a brown recluse, or a tarantula. Follow these steps to treat a spider bite.

1. Seek medical help immediately, either by dialing 911 or by driving to the doctor's office or the emergency room.

2. Have the victim lie down, and keep him or her quiet and warm.

3. Keep the bite area immobile and, if possible, lower than the heart (to slow the speed at which the venom circulates).

4. Wash the bite site with soap and water.

5. If the person who was bitten is not allergic, you can give him or her Tylenol to ease the pain. Be careful when dispensing pain relievers, however. In rare cases, aspirin can actually interfere with the blood's ability to clot and can "conspire" with the venom to spread the injury and make it worse. Your best bet is to give nothing. But if pain is severe, give acetaminophen (Tylenol), which will not do any harm.

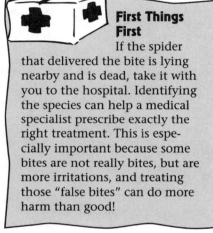

First Things First

If the spider that delivered the bite is lying nearby and is dead, take it with you to the hospital. Identifying the species can help a medical specialist prescribe exactly the right treatment. This is especially important because some bites are not really bites, but are more irritations, and treating those "false bites" can do more harm than good!

6. Tie a strip of cloth, a belt, a watchband, or the sleeve of a shirt two to four inches above the affected area. The bandage should be snug, but loose enough to fit a finger underneath it. (This ensures that you are not completely cutting off the circulation.)

7. If the affected area starts to swell near the strip of cloth, tie another strip two to four inches above the first, and then remove the first strip.

8. Apply ice in a compress or wrapped in a towel or cloth to alleviate the pain. Place the compress over the cloth. (Always wrap the ice before placing it on the bite; plain ice sticks to the skin and causes more irritation.)

9. While you wait for help to arrive, observe the victim for signs of shock or difficulty breathing. (See Chapter 3 for symptoms of and treatment for those conditions.)

Mosquitoes: The Vampires of the Insect World

Only the female of the mosquito species can bite, and she is very particular. Sometimes she will bite only birds or lizards; at other times, she loves certain scents that emanate from humans. If you happen to be one of the "lucky" ones whose perfume or natural scent attracts mosquitoes, you probably already know that, although irritating and uncomfortable, mosquito bites are rarely dangerous.

Here's what happens. The nocturnal female mosquito (after buzzing in your ear and keeping you awake for at least half an hour) finds the perfect spot on your arm. She nestles down on the fleshy arm, and with her *mandibles* and *maxillae* (read: insect jaws and teeth), she literally saws through the skin. When the wound is an appropriate size, she injects saliva into the wound. This keeps your blood from clotting as she sucks it up into her abdomen. Once satisfied, she flies away. The itching you feel after a mosquito bite is the result of the saliva she injects to avoid blood clotting.

Mosquitoes in tropical climates have been known to transmit such diseases as yellow fever, malaria, encephalitis (or sleeping sickness), and filariasis (a disease that affects the lymph glands). These diseases are primarily viruses transmitted through an infected mosquito's saliva, or infections caused by parasites growing within the mosquito (which swim out in the saliva). However, most mosquitoes, especially in America, are more nuisance than danger.

You can take the following preventative measures to cut down on the number of bites you get.

➤ Use an insect repellent such as OFF! when you go outside during the summer months.

➤ Wear a sunscreen that contains mosquito repellent. A good choice is Avon's Skin-So-Soft. (Make sure your bottle has an SPF factor on it; Avon only recently added sunscreen to their product.)

➤ Wear long pants, socks, shoes, and long sleeve T-shirts when roaming through the woods during the summer months.

➤ Avoid perfumes, aftershaves, and scented deodorants during the summer months.

➤ Periodically spray your house and garage with an exterminator "bomb" or repellent at a time when you and your pets will be away for at least five hours. (You should also put your plants on the porch during that time.)

➤ Get inoculations before traveling to the tropics to avoid any diseases transmitted by insects.

First Things First
If you push a mosquito away in the midst of the biting process, you will actually experience more itching! If the mosquito has a chance to finish sucking your blood, much of the saliva she injected during the process will be removed along with the blood.

Ouch!
Unfortunately, some strains of mosquitoes today have become more deadly in the United States. Outbreaks of viral encephalitis (which is transmitted by mosquitoes), have occurred and have resulted in some deaths. The symptoms include temperatures higher than 101 degrees, headache, neck pain, confusion, nausea, and vomiting. If a person exhibits any of these symptoms, take him or her to the emergency room immediately. He or she probably doesn't even remember—or know—that a mosquito bite is to blame!

Chiggers, Bedbugs, Fleas, and Gnats: The Mosquito's Kissing Cousins

Like their mosquito relative, these insects are more annoying than harmful. They do not cause serious diseases in humans except in tropical climes. Preventative measures are basically the same for these as for mosquitoes.

Bedbugs almost look like tiny cockroaches. They are yellow, red, or brown and have a flat oval-shaped body and six legs. You'll find bedbugs in corners, in niches, under wallpaper, and, yes, in dirty, unaired beds. Your best bet to avoid bedbugs? Keep rooms clean and air out your mattresses and mattress pads during spring cleaning time.

Chiggers are just "adorable" with their red or transparent bodies and velvet-like hair on their round bodies. They like damp vegetation and soil like that around your tomato plants and roses. And unfortunately, like lice, they like damp dense hair. There are special shampoos that will kill chiggers and lice in the hair. The main key to dealing with them is to *not* share brushes or combs during the infestation period!

Fleas are the bane of every pet owner's existence. These spry, almost microscopic, brown or black jumpers live in pet hair. Unfortunately, they will also jump to sofas, carpets, and humans if you use a flea repellent on your pet. The only way to get rid of fleas is to use this tried and true three-step process:

1. Flea bomb your house and lawn (carefully following the directions on the container) to avoid re-infestation.

2. Have your pet "dipped" in flea repellent to kill any stray fleas.

3. Wait a week (to let the chemicals "quiet" down). Then use a flea collar or apply flea powder or brewers' yeast (a natural flea repellent) to keep those pesky fleas at bay.

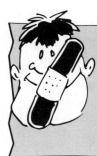

Before You Put the Band-Aid On

Here's a handy hint to further ensure you have a flealess house, pet, and family: add flea powder to your vacuum cleaner bag. If there are some stubborn survivors living on your furniture or your shag rug, they'll be destroyed when they hit the bag. As further prevention, make sure you replace the vacuum bag every time you vacuum in the summer.

Gnats are the most ubiquitous of bugs. Like flies, they are everywhere—wherever you happen to be. They are tiny, dark insects that you can barely see. But as soon as you get that annoying bite, you'll know they're there. Gnats come out during the summer. They, too, love the sunshine and the outdoors. They are not dangerous, but to avoid them, your best bet is to use an insect repellent.

Treating Bites from Mosquitoes and Other Small, Annoying Critters

To treat the irritating bites from mosquitoes, bedbugs, chiggers, fleas, and gnats, follow these steps:

1. Wash the bite site with soap and water.

2. Apply calamine lotion, a paste made of baking soda and water, or cold, wet cloths or compresses to relieve itching.

3. Seek medical assistance if the person displays any of the following side effects:

   A fever within ten days after the bite

   A throbbing pain that begins at the bite site within hours or even days

   Pus, redness, or swelling near the bite site

   Swollen glands

Any of these symptoms can signal a secondary infection. The person should see a medical professional in order to rule out serious diseases or allergies.

Tick Attack

Ticks have received a lot of attention over the past several years. Being the transmitters of such deadly diseases as Rocky Mountain spotted fever and Lyme Disease, ticks are considered Public Enemy Number One in the eyes of many—especially those who live in the Rocky Mountains or in rural areas. Ticks are definitely a nuisance. Although Lyme Disease has become a serious epidemic in certain parts of the country (specifically Northern climes), most ticks are harmless. The key is to make sure that you completely remove any tick that attaches itself to you.

You'll definitely know a tick when you see one (at least when one attaches itself to you). They are tiny and oval in shape, and they have leathery black or dark-brown skin. Unfortunately, they are not easily discernible when in their natural habitat: woods, trees, shrubs, deer, raccoons, and other forest creatures.

Instead of biting, ticks burrow. They dig into your skin head first, and then hang out, contentedly sucking on your blood. Of course, if you see the tick when it is on the surface of the skin but has not yet

Ouch!
Never pull, pinch, tear, or crush a tick that has already embedded itself in the skin. By doing so, you run the risk of removing only the body and not the head, which can lead to infection.

burrowed, you can quickly pick it up with your fingers and crush it dead. However, if the tick has already embedded itself in the skin getting it off of you can be somewhat tricky. Follow these steps to remove the tick:

1. Force the tick to "let go" by covering it completely with Vaseline, rubbing alcohol, or even salad oil or liquor. The oil closes off its breathing holes, and the tick should let go within 30 minutes.

2. Once the tick surrenders, pull it off the skin very carefully with tweezers.

Ticks are usually harmless.

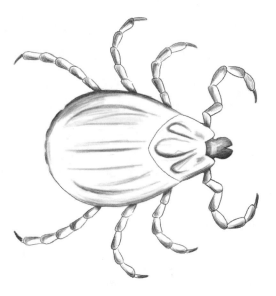

Don't be embarrassed if you'd rather not get rid of the tick on your own. If you are at all fearful of accidentally leaving the head in the skin, take the person to a nearby walk-in or the emergency room for fast, efficient—and safe—removal.

If you wait the full 30 minutes, and the tick refuses to surrender, proceed with these steps:

1. Using tweezers, turn the saturated tick counterclockwise to make it release from the skin, making sure you pick up all its pieces. (It should come out fairly easily because of the oil.)

2. When the tick is out, wash the bite area thoroughly with soap and water.

3. Check for other ticks on the body and scalp.

Signs of Lyme Disease

The spread of Lyme Disease has caused a certain amount of panic, especially among people who live in the Northeast. And statistics add to the scare: 50 percent of the deer ticks found in New Jersey carry Lyme Disease, and raccoons, skunks, mice, and even solid earth itself can hold Lyme-carrying ticks.

The good news is that a blood test can detect Lyme Disease, and antibodies can get rid of it. Even better: scientists have already developed a Lyme Disease vaccine for dogs and cats. It's only a matter of time until we have one as well.

First Aids
Lyme disease gets its name from the town of Lyme, Connecticut, where the first outbreak took place.

If you exhibit any of the following symptoms, see your physician as soon as possible. The presence of these symptoms doesn't mean that you have Lyme Disease; they can indicate other types of infection that might need medical attention.

Swelling of the joints	Swollen glands
Fever within ten days	Throbbing pain at the bite site
Pus oozing from the site	Severe headaches
A red ring-like rash at the bite site within a month	Chronic fatigue

If Lyme Disease is not treated within the first few months, it can infect the heart or nervous system. It can also cause chronic arthritis. If you think you might have been bitten by a tick carrying Lyme Disease, don't hesitate to have a blood test or contact your doctor. It's simple; it's easy; and it will put your mind at ease.

Blood tests are a good way to determine whether or not you have Lyme Disease. But be forewarned. You need to let some time pass (two to three weeks) before taking a test. The results might not show positive for a certain amount of time after the bite. Try to remember when you were bitten and tell your physician. He or she might recommend a second blood test later on if the original test results came back negative but the symptoms continue.

Rocky Mountain "Highs"

Rocky Mountain spotted fever is much less common than Lyme Disease. It is transmitted by a different type of tick that's found mainly in Central and South America, along the eastern coast from Delaware to Florida, and, yes, in the Rocky Mountains.

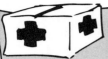

First Things First

Tick prevention is a matter of common sense. Wear long-sleeved shirts, long pants, caps, socks, and shoes when hiking in the woods or vacationing in areas that might be tick-infested. Choose light-colored clothing so that ticks will be more visible on you. Also, spray your campsite with insecticides and inspect each other's skin for ticks at the end of the day. Another plus for insect repellents: they can also keep ticks at bay!

Its initial symptoms are very similar to Lyme Disease, but it will also cause insomnia, restlessness, and some bleeding at the bite site. Symptoms usually occur within two weeks, but if left unchecked, Rocky Mountain spotted fever can cause heart or brain damage. Antibiotics administered in the early stages can eliminate the infection.

Ant Hell

Ants might be small, but they sure know their way around. Ants have inhabited earth for more than 100 million years, and at last count, there were about a quadrillion of them scampering around your picnic grounds and your sugar bowls. Never heard of a quadrillion? That's okay. Just imagine a number that's unimaginable!

Although ants pose a nuisance, they usually don't warrant a first aid call. But some ants do bite. Just ask anyone who has accidentally stepped into a colony of red ants! Symptoms of ant bites include:

Redness at the bite site	Fiery pain
Swelling	Itching

If someone suffers ant bites, administer the first aid outlined in these steps. Ant bites rarely need emergency medical attention.

1. Wash the bite site with soap and cold water

2. Apply calamine lotion or a mixture of baking soda and water

3. If swelling occurs, apply a cold compress or a cold, wet cloth.

First Aids

Although scorpions look like tiny lobsters, these miniature sci-fi creatures are actually members of the same animal group as spiders. These *arachnids* have eight legs, just like spiders, but they have added features: claw-like feelers that they use to grope, and a stinger that paralyzes their prey.

The Deadly Scorpion

Most biologists believe that scorpions were the first animals to crawl out of the sea and decide to live on land. They are nocturnal and tend to live in southwest climes. Believe it or not, scorpions are not aggressive: they would rather run away from a human than fight. Unfortunately, their small shape (only two to three inches long) and brownish-red color (which blends into soil) makes them difficult to see. Many people have been stung by scorpions by simply putting their feet into a pair of shoes that, unbeknownst to them, had been used as a "bed" during the night.

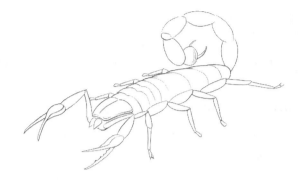

A scorpion can be a deadly enemy.

Symptoms of a scorpion sting include searing pain at the site, nausea, numbness or tingling, fever, stomach cramps, and ultimately convulsions, shock, and inability to speak.

Treating the Suspicious Scorpion Sting

Scorpion stings are dangerous, and they can be deadly. Therefore, they require immediate medical attention. Before help arrives, you can follow these steps for treatment:

1. Have the victim lie down, and if possible, have him keep the affected area still and *lower* than the heart. This slows the rate at which the poison flows through the bloodstream.

2. Wash the site with soap and water.

3. Tie a strip of cloth, a belt, a watchband, or the sleeve of a shirt two to four inches above the affected area. The bandage should be snug, but loose enough to fit a finger underneath it. (This ensures that you are not completely cutting off the circulation.)

4. If the affected area starts to swell near the strip of cloth, tie another strip two to four inches above the first, and then remove the first strip.

5. After 30 minutes, remove the strip. Whatever damage the venom caused will have run its course.

6. Apply ice in a compress or wrapped in a towel or cloth to alleviate the pain. (Always wrap the ice before placing it on the site; plain ice sticks and causes more irritation.)

7. While you wait for help to arrive, watch the victim closely for signs of shock or difficulty breathing. (See Chapter 3 for symptoms and treatments of both.)

A Rash Is a Rash Is a Rash

Rashes can look like raised slashes, red blotches, bumps, or lumps, and they often itch. But if any of the following symptoms is also present, contact a physician. These can signal serious bacterial infections or allergies.

Spots that become bright cherry red or purple

Lumps and bumps that grow bigger and swell

Accompanying fever, nausea, and/or vomiting

Burning and stinging sensations at site

Rashes that suddenly appear while taking new medication

Tenderness or throbbing pain at site

Red streaks leading out from rash to other parts of body

Oozing welts

Swollen glands

A sudden rash could be one of many things. For example, it could be an allergic reaction to a certain medication, the result of contact with poison ivy or some other irritating plant, the result of an insect bite, the effect of a case of nerves (which soon disappears), or a symptom of a serious bacterial infection. The first step in treating a rash is to discover its cause.

Allergies

If the rash doesn't appear to be the result of a bite, you need to determine if it's an allergic reaction. Having a family medical history for each family member (see Chapter 5) can be very helpful at such a time. Consider each of the possible reactions outlined here.

First Aids
Hives are not just homes for bees. A hive is different than a rash because it is raised. Hives are bumps of any size that itch or sting. Desensitizing shots can alleviate hives, and over-the-counter antihistamines can relieve their symptoms.

Medicine: Perhaps the sufferer has developed an allergy to a drug she is taking (such as a sulfur drug she might be taking to treat a urinary tract infection, or a new antibiotic that has just been prescribed). If hives or rashes appear on the stomach or chest while a person is taking a medication, seek immediate medical attention. An allergy to a medicine can be serious, especially if the rash is combined with high fever and flu-like symptoms.

Food and drink: Allergies can flare up quickly, and they can disappear just as fast. Some people get hives every time they eat a strawberry or kiwi fruit. And some unfortunate people develop an itchy rash on their faces or arms after only a few sips of red wine. Food and drink can create allergies, and one of the symptoms of those allergies is skin rashes.

If a certain food or liquid causes problems for you or someone you know, cease and desist! An allergic reaction can become more serious than the rash; along with the rash or hives, a person can develop breathing problems, high fever, convulsions, and/or shock. If food or drink seems to be a problem, your best bet is to make an appointment with an allergist and determine exactly the cause—and the magnitude of the allergy.

> **Ouch!**
> Antibiotics, sulfur drugs, diuretics, and other medications can cause the skin to become very sensitive to light—especially sunlight. The reactions range from blotchy rashes that will eventually fade to serious sunburns. Ask your pharmacist or physician about any medications you are taking.

Fragrances and springtime air: Ah! The scent of spring. The lilacs, the lilies, the intoxicating air of flowers in bloom. Ahh-choo! Unfortunately, when warm weather arrives, many of us experience allergies. Pollen and humidity, and even the perfume found in tissues and magazine ads that mimic flowers and spring can activate allergies and the accompanying sneezes, sniffles, and skin rashes. The good news is that there are medications available to let you breathe deep without side effects, enabling you to enjoy the fragrance of springtime all year long.

Animal life: Many people also suffer from allergies to dogs and cats. Although most people believe it is the fur of these critters that cause rashes and stuffy noses, it is actually the dander that the fur creates (the particles that come in contact with your skin as you pet an animal or that float off an animal's fur into the air). Like dust mites, animal dander inhabits a room even if all you see is a rawhide bone.

Insect bites can also cause allergic reactions and can sometimes have serious results. See the beginning of this chapter for information on bee and wasp allergies.

Poison I-I-I-IVY, Poison I-I-IVEE

Like the old song says, some of the worst skin rashes come from plants and trees. Poison ivy, poison oak, and poison sumac all produce an oily substance that can irritate the skin of most people.

➤ Poison ivy is a green plant that grows low to the ground. It always appears as a shiny cluster of three reddish-green, teardrop-shaped leaves.

➤ Poison oak looks a lot like grape ivy. It is a vine with clusters of three leaves, sometimes three clusters to a branch; all of the leaves are wavy-edged.

➤ Poison sumac is usually found on trees in forests, but it can also grow on a bush. Its leaves are pointed like a palm fan and grow in pairs, except at the tip where there is always one leaf.

Poison ivy, poison oak, and poison sumac can cause severe rashes and itching.

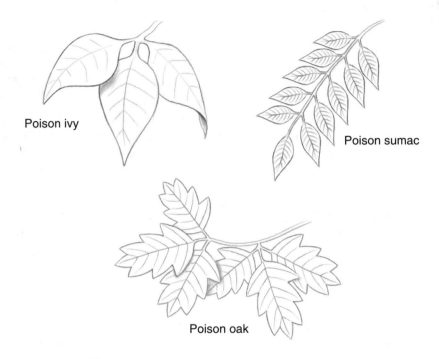

Poison ivy

Poison sumac

Poison oak

Treating Poison Ivy and Its "Cousins"

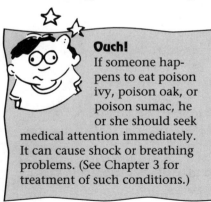

Ouch!
If someone happens to eat poison ivy, poison oak, or poison sumac, he or she should seek medical attention immediately. It can cause shock or breathing problems. (See Chapter 3 for treatment of such conditions.)

Symptoms of the irritation caused by the three poison plants include red rashes (sometimes accompanied by small blisters), itching, possible headache and fever, and a blistering rash. Coming into contact with poison ivy, poison oak, or poison sumac is rarely fatal. In fact, it does not require professional help—unless a person suffers a severe allergic reaction.

However, it's important to treat symptoms from poison ivy and its cousins because it can spread to other parts of the body. It can even spread from clothes to skin. Follow these steps:

1. Take off all clothes that have come in contact with the poisonous plant and wash them in hot water.

2. Wash any part of the skin (especially where a rash appears) that might have come in contact with contaminated clothes or the plant itself. Use soap and hot water.

3. Wipe the skin with a cotton ball, a tissue, or a washcloth dipped in alcohol.

4. Apply calamine lotion to relieve discomfort and itching.

Prickly Heat

These tiny patches of red dots don't just appear on babies' bottoms. Chafing, too much sweating from exercise or heat, or a lack of proper clothing ventilation can cause prickly heat, which is caused by blocked sweat glands. The best treatment is to wear loose, light clothes in hot weather. You can also use powder to avoid chafing.

> **Ouch!**
> If a poisonous plant comes into contact with the mouth or the genitals, it's important to seek medical help. Any contamination on the mouth can result in breathing problems, and any contamination on the genitals can cause urinary irritation.

Other Skin Problems

No we're not talking about blackheads, pimples, acne scars, or wrinkles. However unpleasant they might look, pimples and laugh lines are no threat to your life (unless, of course, you are a supermodel!). But some skin irritations signal allergies or bacterial infections that can be serious. In order to be able to help someone, you must be able to recognize the kind of skin problem you are dealing with and determine whether you need to seek emergency medical care.

Psoriasis is a skin problem that you can thank your parents (or grandparents) for; it's an inherited condition. It creates a scaly, peeling rash that can be treated with medication. It rarely occurs as a result of improper hygiene or sanitation.

Athlete's Foot is a fungus that usually occurs between the toes. It creates a scaly, moist, itchy rash that can be treated with antifungal creams and powders available at any drugstore. It usually becomes worse when one doesn't dry properly between the toes. (Remember what your mother said!)

Eczema is a superficial inflammation of the skin that is usually caused by irritations from detergents, soaps, and cleaners. Cortisone creams can relieve the symptoms of scaly, itchy, flaky redness. You can now purchase prescription-strength cortisone creams over-the-counter in your drugstore.

Impetigo is an infection of the skin caused by staph or strep bacteria (the same germs that cause colds and sore throats). It creates pus-filled bumps and scaly blisters that eventually break and crust. Medical attention is essential for impetigo because it can spread to other parts of the body and to other people. Antibiotics will get rid of the bacteria. In addition, it's important to wash all clothes, towels, and bedding that might be contaminated in hot water.

The Least You Need to Know

➤ Bees and wasps have different stings, but both can cause an allergic reaction. Symptoms include gasping for breath, a flushed face, and an inability to swallow. It should be treated as a crisis medical emergency. Seek help fast!

➤ There are only three types of poisonous spiders: the black widow, the brown recluse, and the tarantula. However, none of those usually cause a fatal reaction. Symptoms of one of their bites include profuse sweating, nausea and stomach cramps, difficulty breathing, and a tingling sensation in the body. Keep the person prone, quiet, and warm. Wash the affected area with soap and water.

➤ Your pets (and maybe you, someday) can be vaccinated against Lyme Disease, a condition caused by a deer tick. Symptoms of Lyme Disease include arthritic aches and pains, chronic fatigue, and memory loss.

➤ Mosquitoes can be more dangerous than you think. Some types carry serious diseases such as malaria and encephalitis. If someone you know suddenly gets an abrupt high fever over 101 degrees, accompanied by headache, neck pain, confusion, nausea, and vomiting, get him or her to the emergency ward immediately.

➤ If you happen to be in the Southwest, don't ever put on a pair of shoes without checking the insides. A scorpion might be sleeping in one of them!

➤ Treat scorpion bites by keeping the person in a prone position, washing the bitten area with soap and water, and applying a very loose tourniquet. Check those ABCs of first aid regularly: make sure Airways are clear, Breathing is regular, and Circulation is normal.

➤ You need to be able to recognize the three types of plants (poison ivy, poison sumac, and poison oak) that secrete an oil that causes rashes. Symptoms of contact with one of these plants include a rash, itching, and possible headaches and fever. Such contact is rarely life-threatening unless the leaves are swallowed.

➤ The most dangerous skin problems are those caused by bacteria and some allergies. Impetigo, for example, is caused by bacteria and is treated with antibiotics. Check with your pharmacist and doctor to verify that the medications you are taking will not have any side-effects from sunlight (causing rashes or severe sunburn).

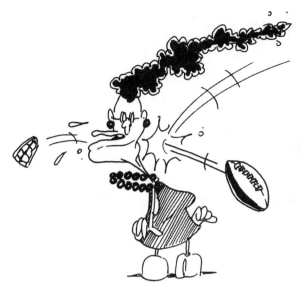

Chapter 20

Mouth and Tooth Injuries

In This Chapter

➤ Dealing with the universal mouth ailment: a toothache

➤ Handling a loose tooth or tooth injury

➤ Putting a stop to bleeding gums and tissue

➤ Easing pain from dentures or braces

Almost everyone, at one time or another, has been through the unpleasant experience of a toothache. In the olden days, this meant pulling out the aching tooth with a black-smith tool or a wrench—and without benefit of anesthesia to ease the pain! The alcohol given to dental sufferers in those days probably did more to ward off infection than to numb the pain. And infections were common, sometimes moving from tooth to tooth along the gum line. The result? An attractive mouth full of wooden dentures.

In the modern world, mouth and tooth problems are taken care of with much less pain and discomfort. But to avoid infection, it's good to know what to do if a tooth suddenly falls out, if a child gets hit in the mouth with a ball, or if braces are causing mouth irritations. The first aid care described in this chapter can help you deal with mouth pain until you can make that visit to the dreaded "D" word: the dentist.

The Universal, Age-Old Complaint: a Toothache

There's not much you can do for a toothache except go to a dentist. A toothache is not a life-threatening condition, but it sure can feel like one. Ouch!

A toothache is often like appendicitis: it hits you hard all at once. Basically, a tooth starts to ache because it has become infected and inflamed, which puts pressure on the nerve of the tooth or the ligaments in the gum that keeps teeth in your mouth. In reality, that sudden pain could have been years in the making.

There are several reasons why a tooth starts to ache, including:

Years of sloppy dental care (such as improper brushing and lack of flossing teeth)

A broken filling

Recent dental work

A cracked tooth

A popcorn kernel (or other food) that's stuck under the gum line

Obviously, the popcorn kernel represents the easiest toothache to fix. The others might need more care—especially those that result from poor dental hygiene. Toothaches caused by improper care can mean that decay and its accompanying infection has reached the point where it has struck the nerve. Although the pain might eventually go away, it will come back. And the next time, it will be with an abscess that's filled with pus and a swollen jaw.

In many cases, unless the toothache is caused by something as minor as a popcorn kernel or a loose filling, it is a signal that the tooth must come out. This doesn't have to fill you with fear. Dentists today are very sensitive to the fact that many patients are terrified. Not only are there local anesthetics to numb the affected area, but a good dentist will explain what is going on, step-by-step, so you are not sitting there helpless and feeling left in the dark.

But what if the dentist can't see you right away? Here are some tips to keep pain from getting worse while you wait:

1. Take ibuprofen, an anti-inflammatory pain reliever. Because a toothache is caused by inflammation, medications such as Advil and Motrin can reduce swelling, which consequently relieves the pressure on the tooth nerve.

2. Place an ice pack on the cheek or chin, wherever the pain is most severe. It can help numb the ache. But don't chew crushed ice! It can break teeth and cause another toothache!

A Child's Loose Tooth

There are times when a loose tooth is perfectly normal. Losing teeth is a rite of passage: baby teeth fall out, and adult teeth begin to peek through the gums.

The tooth fairy's surprise aside, losing a baby tooth rarely causes any complications. But sometimes a loose tooth refuses to come out on its own. In that case, you can carefully pull it yourself. If a child's tooth moves back and forth easily without pain, follow these steps to pull it:

1. Wash your hands thoroughly with soap and water.

2. Ask your child to open wide. Try to keep him or her calm. The anticipated tooth fairy's visit is always a good fear reliever!

3. Using a clean gauze pad, gently pull the tooth out with your fingers.

4. The gum above the removed tooth might bleed. If so, have the child lean slightly forward to avoid swallowing any blood (and becoming nauseated).

5. Using a new gauze pad, apply pressure to the gum area until bleeding stops.

6. Bleeding should stop within a few minutes. If, after fifteen minutes, the bleeding continues, seek professional medical help.

7. (Optional) Put the tooth under the child's pillow before he or she goes to sleep so the tooth fairy will visit!

Ouch!
Be sure to check the area where the tooth has been removed to make sure no tooth fragments are left behind. Especially if a tooth is knocked out, fragments are very possible, and the victim should visit a dentist as soon as possible.

Losing Caps or Dentures

Just as children lose their baby teeth, adults can lose an implanted cap or a piece of a denture. Caps are usually glued with the intent that they will stay for many, many years. But in the event that one falls off, you should see your dentist as soon as possible. Exposed tooth pulp tissue can be very susceptible to infection and very painful. (And of course, we won't mention the lovely look of a broken front cap!)

It is not necessary to rinse your mouth with an antiseptic. Dentists recommend that you buy "tooth adhesive," which can be purchased over the counter in drugstores to keep a tooth in place until your appointment. It can help keep the area from being exposed—and it will look a whole lot better than a gaping hole.

When a piece of a denture breaks, it's important to see your dentist. The broken off crown, implant, or cap has been acting as a type of shield, covering and protecting the gum line from exposure. Without that piece of denture, the gum is vulnerable to infection.

Treating Cuts and Bleeding on Lips or Gums

Rarely are cuts and scrapes on or in the mouth an emergency. You should expect bleeding—but do not be alarmed! Direct pressure on the spot that's cut will usually stop the bleeding within minutes.

Ouch!
Most cuts on the lips or gums are caused by items that are fairly clean, such as eating utensils, toothbrushes, or dental floss. But if a dirty foreign object hits the mouth—say, a fist, a tennis ball, or a paw that's been tromping through mud— it's best to go see your medical professional. If you've not received a tetanus shot in the past 10 years, you might need one to ward off disease.

To stop any bleeding in the mouth, you should use the following general first aid steps:

1. Always wash out the injured person's mouth with cool water to remove any dirt. (And always wash your hands first in soap and water!)

2. Have the victim lean slightly forward to keep blood from draining back into the throat and causing nausea.

3. Using a sterile gauze pad, apply direct pressure on the cut site.

4. If the cut is on the lip, hold the lip with the gauze pad in both hands. Press hard on both the outside and the inside of the lip.

Apply direct pressure to the mouth to stop bleeding.

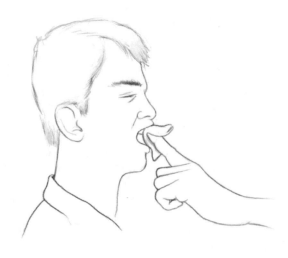

Braces can make a hit, a fall, or a slam on the mouth much more painful. Braces can get caught on the lip or the mouth, and the dented metal can bruise the inside of the cheek. Although braces are made of materials much gentler than the "metal barbed wire" of yore, they can still do damage. The best bet is to treat bleeding with salt water to ward off infection. Then hold a gauze pad over the wound to staunch bleeding if necessary. (The pad will also act as padding.) Take the victim to the orthodontist or a walk-in medical center as soon as possible.

Follow these steps to soothe an irritated or bleeding tongue:

> **First Things First**
> Believe it or not, one of the best ways to stop bleeding gums is with a tea bag. The tannic acid in the tea helps constrict blood vessels and makes for faster clotting. Simply use a teabag instead of a gauze pad.

1. Pull the tongue out and press the gauze pad on both sides with two fingers.

2. If, perhaps, the tongue is irritated from food that's too hot, apply some ice in a cloth after the bleeding stops.

3. For a severe burn of the tongue, seek emergency help immediately.

To treat bleeding gums or tooth sockets, place a gauze pad on the site that is bleeding and irritated. Press hard with your fingers (but not so hard that you cause more pain!).

Managing Injuries to the Jaw

If someone gets hit in the jaw (or, in the PG-rated version, if he inadvertently falls on the ground), not only does it hurt, but the jaw can be misaligned or broken. The best thing to do in the event of a jaw injury is to get medical help as soon as possible. Either call 911 or drive the victim to the hospital emergency room. Only a physician can determine if a jaw is broken, misaligned, or merely bruised. A misaligned jaw can cause chewing problems as well as muscle and bone complications. You can treat the jaw injury in the following ways to ease the discomfort until a professional can take a look at it.

➤ Apply a cold compress or ice wrapped in a cloth.

➤ Treat bleeding with gentle pressure only, and wash away blood if it accumulates.

➤ Do not touch, open, or manipulate the mouth in any way unless it's absolutely necessary.

Knocked-Out Teeth

In addition to bleeding profusely, a suddenly empty tooth socket can cause serious pain and become infected, especially if particles of the pulp or root remain. If you have a tooth knocked out, get to a dentist immediately. (If that's not possible, call 911 or drive yourself to the emergency room.) If possible, take the tooth with you. If you can get yourself and the tooth to a dentist within a couple of hours, there's a good chance that the dentist will be able to successfully reimplant the tooth.

Until you can get to the dentist, keep the tooth wrapped in a strip of clean, wet gauze. Place a clean, sterile gauze pad on the empty socket and press down on the pad. This helps keep bleeding under control.

Embracing Braces

Orthodontics might not be the prettiest site to behold, but when they are finally removed, they create beautifully aligned teeth that will stay healthy for years to come. Today's braces are a far cry from the "barbaric" metal clips and wires of yesteryear, the glinting, reflecting steel that made many a high school student refuse to open her mouth in the yearbook picture.

Now you can give a smile as big as Julia Robert's trademark, thanks to braces that are transparent or that match your tooth color. Further, braces are now used at a bare minimum; sometimes only the teeth that really need them are wrapped in a band. And some people only have to wear braces at night—which means that if you're single, no one ever has to know you visit a (ssshh!) orthodontist.

Even with all these advances, braces can still irritate the gums, the roof of the mouth, the cheeks, and the tongue. Only your orthodontist can rearrange the braces to prevent irritation and pressure. But while you're waiting for the appointment, there are several things you can do to ease the pain.

> ➤ Place a cotton ball or a folded up gauze pad over the offending wire.

> ➤ Take aspirin or some other pain reliever to ease the pain.

> ➤ Gargle with warm salt water to prevent infection and provide relief.

The Least You Need to Know

> ➤ If a tooth falls out, make sure no fragments or pulp are left behind.

> ➤ Bleeding in the mouth is easily remedied with clean hands, a clean gauze pad, and direct pressure.

> ➤ Always try to find the tooth that's been knocked out. They can often be reimplanted within two hours of the accident.

> ➤ Jaw injuries *always* require medical attention.

> ➤ Although only an orthodontist can fix braces, you can relieve the pain while you wait for an appointment. Warm salt water, over the counter pain relievers, and gauze pads can all help.

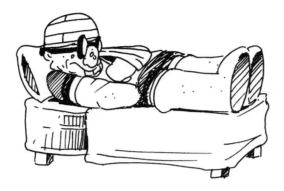

Chapter 21

Muscle Cramps, Strains, Sprains, and Breaks

In This Chapter

➤ Treating cramps, strains, and sprains: do you apply heat or cold?

➤ When a muscle cramp can signal something dangerous

➤ Sprains versus breaks

A muscle cramp can be caused by something as trivial as gas. On the other hand, it can be a symptom of appendicitis—or even a heart attack. Likewise, a strain can be the result of being at the gym a half hour too long, but it can ultimately lead to inflamed muscles and painful pinched nerves.

Sprains and breaks, too, can be simple to handle—or the start of something complicated. Obviously, a broken bone must be treated properly for correct alignment as it heals. But a sprain is more subtle. It might require an Ace bandage and staying off your feet for a day or two—or, without the right treatment, it can lead to swelling and pain and (eventually) chronic nerve, muscle, or bone damage and arthritis.

But never fear. By the time you finish reading this chapter, you will know how to differentiate these conditions, how to treat them, and how to prevent them from occurring in the first place.

Cramping Your Style: Muscle Cramps and Strains

A muscle cramp can be one of the fallouts of exercise, especially on hot days. Suppose for example, the muscle in your arm or leg suddenly—and painfully—knots itself into a tight fist. Cramps can also occur when you move around in bed or even when you're simply taking a nap.

A muscle strain is more serious, especially when it affects the muscles in the back. A strain involves injury not only to muscles, but also to ligaments, tendons, or blood vessels surrounding a bone joint. The injured tissue is either pulled, stretched, wrenched, or torn during physical activity (like when you took that flying leap across the room during your first dance class in thirty years!).

Treating Muscle Cramps

Muscle cramps are easy to fix and do not require emergency first aid. Treat them in this way:

1. Stretch out the muscle as soon as you feel a cramp.

2. Massage the knotted muscle with the heel of the hand for several minutes.

3. Follow the massage with a warm bath, warm wet compresses, or a heating pad to provide soothing heat. This should release the knot.

Muscle cramps commonly affect the calf or the heel of the foot during exercise or team sports. If this happens to someone you're with, have him or her perform a forward stretch in which the cramped leg leans forward and the cramped foot is flat on the floor (as shown in the following illustration). Then massage the cramp while in this position.

Stretch and massage cramped calves.

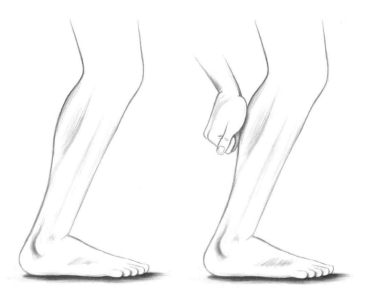

196

Treating Muscle Strains

You treat muscle strains by doing the exact opposite of what you would do for a cramp.

➤ Do not stretch or massage the muscle; instead keep it at rest.

➤ Elevate a strained arm or leg to prevent swelling.

➤ Think *cold*: place cold wet cloths or a cold compress on the muscle. The appropriate technique for "icing" an injury is to wrap ice in a clean cloth and alternately apply the ice to the injury for 20 minutes, remove the ice for 20 minutes, and reapply (with fresh ice) for 20 minutes. Repeat this cycle for the first full day. You need to keep the muscle cold for the first 24 hours to prevent the muscle fiber from swelling, which could touch a nerve and cause even more pain.

➤ After 24 hours, turn to warmth: use hot wet compresses to soothe the muscle. The warmth increases blood circulation and aids faster healing.

➤ Ibuprofen can help ease the pain and reduce inflammation.

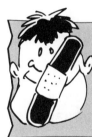

Before You Put the Band-Aid On

Cramps and strains require different treatment. So how can you tell the difference between the two? A cramp hurts less, and the pain is usually more localized. A strain causes severe pain and possible swelling.

Warning Signs of Other Conditions

A muscle cramp can be a result of too much exercise or a sudden wrong move, but it can also signal too much stress—or worse. If any cramp keeps coming back, it could be a warning sign of a serious disease. Check with your physician.

When your *neck and shoulders* cramp up, it's a good idea to stop what you are doing, roll your head from side-to-side, and shrug your shoulders. Relaxation exercises and meditation can also help this side effect of stress.

When your *stomach* cramps, it can signal gastric distress or even appendicitis. And as your mother used to warn you, stomach cramps in the water can be serious. Although you don't necessarily get a stomach cramp if you go swimming after a meal, if they do occur, you could lose control and drown.

Strains, too, can lead to more serious situations. A strained back can leave you incapacitated for days—or weeks. Sometimes simple strains are combined with broken bones. And a severe strain might signal internal bleeding and swelling. If a strain doesn't go away after you follow the basic first aid treatment, see a physician.

Sprains and Breaks

You see children with broken arms or fingers much more often than you do adults. It's a good thing, too. Bones get more brittle with age. An adult's broken arm would take longer to heal, and it might lead to chronic pain. Besides, adults rarely consider getting autographs on a cast "fun." But ask most children about a broken arm or leg, and they will proudly show you colorful, graffiti-covered casts (that are usually gray with dirt).

Whether it happens to a child or an adult, a sprain or a fracture can be serious. Depending on its location, a broken bone can be life-threatening. It can lead to shock, a weak pulse, or breathing difficulties. And at the very least, a sprain or break hurts—a lot.

The steps you take to treat a sprain or break until you can get professional care can make the difference in whether a break heals correctly and in proper alignment. It might determine, for example, whether a nose will be permanently out of joint (excuse the expression).

The Differences Between Sprains and Breaks

How are sprains and breaks different? Not by much. A sprain is kind of like a strain at the bone itself; its muscle fibers, connective tissues, or ligaments have been stretched to the max or wrenched completely out of whack.

As you might guess, a break goes one step further: the bone actually breaks. In fact, a break doesn't have to occur only at muscle junctures, such as the elbow or ankle. Bones can break anywhere along their mass, from lower arms to upper thighs, from buttocks and hips to collar bones.

Only with an x-ray can you definitely tell whether a bone is broken. Because sprains and breaks can look similar, you should treat a sprain as if it were a break, and you should have it x-rayed. It's better to be safe than sorry.

Signs of bone injury or joint sprain include:

> Feeling or hearing an actual "snap"
>
> Bluish discoloration or bruising over injured bone or joint
>
> Abnormal position of limb
>
> Inability to move a limb on one's own
>
> Excessive pain at injury site
>
> Swelling, numbness, and tingling near injured bone or joint

Broken Bones: The Four Fs

A broken bone is called a fracture. There are four types of fractures:

➤ A *simple* fracture (also called a closed fracture) is when the bone breaks cleanly in two. The skin remains intact and unbroken, and all the damage is internal.

➤ A *compound* (or open) fracture is a fracture in which the skin is most definitely broken, either from an object that pierces the skin and breaks the bone within, or from a part of the broken bone itself that pushes out through the skin. Treat any bleeding from the open wound by gently wiping it away with a clean cloth.

➤ A *comminuted* fracture has multiple breaks in one bone. These breaks can be simple or compound (they may or may not pierce the skin).

➤ A *green stick* fracture is a "young" break that doesn't go straight through the bone (similar to a young green tree branch that doesn't break completely in two). This type of fracture usually occurs in children because their bones are not yet mature and firm.

> **Ouch!**
> Never give a person with a broken bone anything to eat or drink or any medication to swallow. It can cause nausea and blockage, which can further damage the injured area or cause breathing problems.

The Joys of Ace Bandages

These versatile elastic strips of flesh-colored cloth are best for problems in small places: ankles, wrists, feet, and hands. As a matter of fact, they are perfect for keeping small areas immobile, aligned, and comfortable.

To use an Ace bandage, simply place one end of the bandage on, say, the ankle. Holding that end in place with one hand, use your other hand to wrap the bandage around the ankle and around the foot, turning and turning, until it is secure. (You can remove your first hand when the wrap becomes stable.)

> **Ouch!**
> Using an Ace bandage on an arm, leg, or shoulder can inhibit circulation and cause the same heart and circulation problems that a tourniquet can.

You secure the bandage in place with the two clips that come with it. These clips have tiny hooks that slip into the bandage itself wherever you want to place them. They are much more convenient and safe than safety pins and much more secure than tape.

Ace bandages are ideal for wrapping ankles.

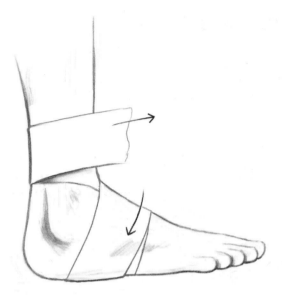

Treating Sprains and Breaks

There are four basic rules when it comes to "dem bones" first aid:

➤ Get the injured person to an emergency treatment location as soon as possible.

➤ Keep the injured area immobile to prevent further injury and excessive pain.

➤ While you are waiting, watch the person's vital signs (those ABCs: Airways clear, Breathing regular, Circulation steady). You do not want the injured person to go into shock (see Chapter 3).

➤ Remember: There is very little you can do to repair broken bones or tissue damage. You can only make waiting a little easier.

Bandaging sprains and breaks to keep injured arms, legs, shoulders, feet, and hands immobile is an important part of the waiting game. Using Ace bandages, splints, and slings, you can do a very competent job of keeping the injury status quo. Chapter 4 contains step-by-step instructions for bandaging different parts of the body.

Dislocation

No, this doesn't mean you are lost at sea or on the road. Dislocation means that a bone or piece of cartilage at a joint actually becomes displaced. The round parts of bones fit into sockets, like a foot fits snugly into a sock. If one of these pieces is pushed slightly askew, it can cause tremendous, immediate, and extreme pain.

Dislocations are particularly common in shoulders, hips, knees, and fingers. In toddlers, the most common dislocations are at the elbow, when a child is being swung by her arms in play or she is inadvertently lifted by one arm. Dislocations can be especially dangerous to children because their bones are still growing and a dislocation can actually affect the way the bones develop.

If a dislocation occurs, the person's limb will be at an odd angle. And they will almost undoubtedly be screaming out in pain because dislocation causes extreme pain! Administer first aid for a dislocation by following these guidelines:

➤ Get to an emergency room fast. An experienced physician can usually "slip" the joint back into place fairly easily.

➤ To help ease the pain and facilitate transport, use bandages to wrap the injured limb in a way that will ease some of the pain by taking pressure off of it. A loose bandage will also keep the bone from moving away from the socket more. (For example, a bandage used as a sling can help prevent further injury to a dislocated shoulder.)

➤ Apply an ice pack to the area to numb the pain.

> **Ouch!**
> Even if you've seen someone else put a dislocated joint back into place, don't try it on your own (unless, maybe, you are miles from civilization). You can end up making the dislocation—and the pain—much worse.

The Least You Need to Know

➤ Sprains and strains, broken bones, and cramps are a part of life—especially if you or your family members are active and physical. These injuries are rarely life-threatening (unless damage occurs to the head or back—or to the hip in the elderly).

➤ A cramp is the mildest of muscle problems. Unless the cramp occurs repeatedly in a short period of time, it's nothing to worry about. To treat a cramp, apply massage and heat.

➤ A strain is exactly what it sounds like: a muscle that is stretched to the limits. Use cold compresses for a strain.

➤ The best first aid for fractures and sprains is simple: keep the status quo. Make the injured person comfortable, and keep the injured site immobile.

➤ Anytime someone suffers what might be a fracture or a sprain, he should have the injury x-rayed just to be sure.

➤ Never try to force a dislocated bone back into place. Wait for help.

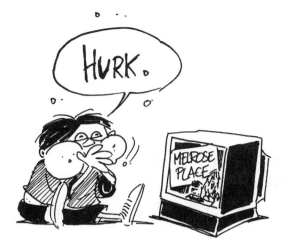

Nausea, Vomiting, and Food Poisonings

Purging was *de riguer* in medicine until the nineteenth century. Ill people were frequently given a vile-tasting concoction that would force them to vomit, purging them of whatever sickness they were suffering from. Obviously, purging wasn't a success all (or most) of the time, but it is still a method of choice to get rid of certain poisons. And as every cat knows, it's a great way to get rid of hairballs.

Nausea and vomiting go together, in not quite as mundane a fashion as socks and shoes, but a combination nonetheless. In fact, when you are nauseated, vomiting frequently gets rid of the problem.

However, nausea and vomiting are not always paired. Nausea can signal a gastrointestinal problem, fever, or a flu. Vomiting can result from food poisoning or overindulgence. And excessive vomiting can create such problems as airway blockage, dehydration, and shock.

Step-by-Step First Aid for Minor Upsets

Even without that nauseous "I can't believe I ate the whole thing" feeling, vomiting is extremely common. It can be the result of too much food or drink, a minor flu, motion sickness, emotional stress, an allergy, or a side effect to medication.

A minor upset is basically vomiting or nausea that lasts no longer than a day (often called a "24-hour bug"), or vomiting or nausea without other such symptoms as fever, severe abdominal pain, blood in the vomit, or chills.

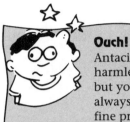

Ouch!
Antacids seem harmless enough, but you should always read the fine print before administering them to a person who's ill. Certain over-the-counter medications can cause allergic reactions if mixed with antibiotics, antidepressants, or other medication.

Treat a minor stomach upset in the following way:

1. Immediately cut all solid foods from the ill person's diet.

2. Give the ill person an over-the-counter medicine for acid indigestion or nausea, either in liquid form, chewable tablets, or tablets that dissolve in water.

These two steps might be all you need to stop the symptoms. But if vomiting (with or without nausea) occurs for several more hours, continue with these first aid steps:

1. Because dehydration can occur after several hours of vomiting, you should replace lost fluids with bland, clear beverages, either hot or cold. These can include tea, chicken broth, apple juice, ginger ale, clear colas, and (that old standby) water. (Ginger ale and cola are especially good for settling queasy stomachs.)

2. If the ill person begins to feel better and stops vomiting, add bland solid foods to the diet. Plain toast, crackers, and farina are all good choices.

When Vomiting Is More Than Just Gross: The Danger Signs

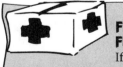

First Things First
If an ill person loses consciousness but is still vomiting, turn his or her head to the side to prevent choking and airway blockage.

Mild vomiting accompanied by nausea is something we've all experienced at one time or another. But if a person has any of the following symptoms in combination with vomiting, emergency aid is crucial:

Unconsciousness

Continuous stabbing pain, especially in the abdominal area

Dizziness

Stomach bloating

Headaches

Prolonged vomiting

Fever and chills

Bloody vomit

Any of these symptoms can signal more serious conditions, such as appendicitis, food poisoning, hernia complications, intestinal blockage, and even drug overdose.

With severe vomiting, the first and foremost first aid step is to get help as fast as you can. If you have a vehicle at your disposal, rush the victim to the nearest emergency ward (with the window open!) or dial 911. This condition requires medical attention immediately! In addition to that, follow these guidelines:

➤ Do not administer any beverages or medications.

➤ Keep the ill person as comfortable as possible until help arrives. Cover him or her with a loose blanket, apply a soothing cloth to his or her forehead, and wipe the mouth and chin as necessary.

➤ Watch the person's vital signs and take charge if there is any change in circulation, pulse, or breathing (see Chapter 3).

Food Poisoning

We've all read reports about undercooked chicken and pork, mayonnaise and eggs left out in the sun too long, seafood that's gone from overripe to bad. What changes these foods from delicious delights to dangerous disasters? Bacteria, that's what.

Bacteria can cause food poisoning in three ways:

➤ Bacteria that you ingest (in undercooked chicken, for example) can infect the stomach lining.

➤ Bacteria can create toxins in certain foods (such as mayonnaise left outside), and you ingest the toxins.

➤ Bacteria that you ingest (in eggs, for example) can produce toxins after they reach the stomach.

The end result of all of these is nausea, vomiting, chills, and extreme discomfort.

When food is left out in the sun, when meats are not cooked through, or when fish spoils, they become breeding grounds for organisms from bacteria to parasites. As Table 23.1 shows, food gone bad is bacteria's heaven—and our poison hell.

Table 23.1 Food Poisons at a Glance

Type of Bacteria	Cause	Delay Time Before Illness
Staphylococcus	Spoiled foods	A few hours
Salmonella	Undercooked foods	Eight or more hours
Botulinum	Badly canned foods	One or two days

The following sections cover these three common types of bacteria in greater detail.

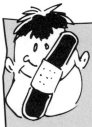

Before You Put the Band-Aid On

There are three less common food poisonings that can pack a deadly wallop. These include:

Escherichia coli: the culprit behind an outbreak of flu-like symptoms and even death that resulted from eating undercooked fast food burgers.

Bacillus cereus: a contamination often associated with fried rice!

Vibrio parahaemocyticus: a poisoning that results from bad seafood, especially shellfish.

All three of these food poisonings require a trip to the emergency room or the family doctor. Side effects include nausea, chills, flu-like symptoms, and even death.

Staphylococcus

It might sound like a mouthful—and it is. The most common type of food poisoning is named from the bacteria that contaminates foods such as mayonnaise left out in the sun, cream or custards that are not fresh, soured milk, and unrefrigerated meats. Those foods provide prime growing ground for the staphylococcus bacteria.

Symptoms of this type of bacterial poisoning will occur almost immediately or within only a few hours. They include nausea and vomiting, diarrhea, stomach pain, and weakness.

The best treatment for staphylococcal poisoning is patience. The symptoms will usually clear up (and out) within a few hours. During that time, make sure the ill person is comfortable and near a bathroom. Do not give him or her any pills or medication, but you can give water if it's requested.

Salmonella

Despite its name, salmonella doesn't just occur in salmon. It too is a bacteria—a more serious cousin to staphylococcus. Salmonella poisoning occurs in contaminated foods, which might or might not be cooked. It is also linked to poor sanitary conditions. (In other words, avoid food stores swarming with insects, heat, and cooks with dirty hands.)

Symptoms of salmonella poisoning usually surface about eight hours after a person eats the bad food. The symptoms are very similar to those of staphylococcal poisoning, but they are much more severe. They include:

Ouch!
Salmonella bacteria is most prevalent in undercooked or improperly cleaned or stored poultry, pork, beef, and eggs.

> Nausea and vomiting
>
> Fever
>
> Chills
>
> Severe diarrhea and abdominal cramps
>
> Flu-like symptoms

If you think someone might have salmonella poisoning, seek medical help immediately. Then make the person as comfortable as possible. Give him or her only water if requested.

Botulinum

The most devious food poisoning, botulism, is also the most deadly. It is an illness caused by the botulinum bacteria. Symptoms usually don't appear until two days after ingestion—and it can sometimes be difficult to trace back to the contaminated food. Botulism is caused by contamination of canned goods; the botulinum bacteria thrives on improperly packaged food and food that is used after it has "turned bad." New studies are also revealing that botulism can occur in gourmet hand-flavored bottled oils, in which whole slivers of peppers or herbs are placed in a glass bottle along with the cooking oil.

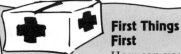

First Things First

How can you tell if the food in a can might have been contaminated? If a can is battered, swollen at the top or bottom, or sold after the "best used by" date, or if it exudes a strong odor when it's opened, you can bet it's probably bad. You should live by the old saying, "When in doubt, throw it out!"

Botulinum bacteria produces symptoms all its own:

Blurriness or dim vision

Double vision

Heavy eyelids

Difficulty breathing

Severe fatigue

Inability to swallow

Garbled speech

If any of these symptoms occur, seek medical assistance immediately. Try to retrace the ill person's routine over the past two days and find the culprit. Finding the food can help the emergency team provide the correct treatment. If the ill person cannot remember what she consumed or if she is too sick to talk, check her appointment book, call her office, and look in the garbage can.

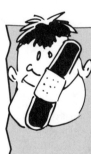

Before You Put the Band-Aid On

The more acidic the canned food is, the less likely the chance that botulinum bacteria can grow in it. The acid kills the enemy before it has time to get a "podhold." Thus most canned goods containing tomatoes (such as tomato soup, stewed tomatoes, tomato sauce, and tomato juice) are probably going to be safe.

The Least You Need to Know

➤ Vomiting and/or nausea is most often caused by overeating, too much alcohol, emotional stress, or motion sickness. A mild case of vomiting usually clears up within 24 hours.

➤ Treat mild cases with over-the-counter medications. (Be sure to read the fine print and make sure the patient isn't taking another medicine that could cause an allergic reaction.) Also for mild cases, provide hot or cold liquids, and then slowly add bland food as the person starts to feel better.

➤ Signs of a more serious problem include blood in the vomit, fever and chills, headaches, severe abdominal pain, and prolonged vomiting.

➤ Serious vomiting, with or without nausea, requires immediate medical attention. This means a visit to the emergency ward, either by calling 911 or driving the victim yourself. Prevent the patient from taking in any liquids or medication until help arrives.

➤ When food spoils, it is a breeding ground for many organisms—from parasites to bacteria—that can make you sick.

➤ Staphylococcus bacteria produces toxins that cause the most common type of food poisoning. It is usually not serious, and patience is all you need to ride out the storm of nausea and vomiting.

➤ Salmonella poisoning usually doesn't show up for approximately eight hours. It usually results from eating undercooked foods, and symptoms include nausea and vomiting. If salmonella poisoning is suspected, take the victim to his or her doctor or the local walk-in medical center.

➤ Botulism is the most serious food poisoning. Sometimes its symptoms, such as nausea and vomiting, don't show up for as much as two days. Other far more serious symptoms include blurred vision, confusion, and garbled speech. This type of food poisoning requires professional medical treatment.

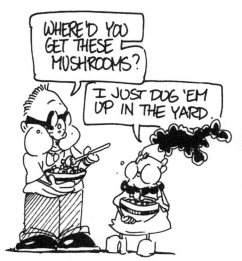

Chapter 23

Poisoning and Drug Overdoses

In This Chapter

➤ Common poisons in the home: cleaning products, food, pesticides, and drugs

➤ Vomiting as a form of treatment

➤ Carbon monoxide: the invisible poison

➤ First aid for drug overdoses

Poison, poison everywhere. Unfortunately, it's in forms that you might drink, inhale, apply, or eat! Toddlers get their hands on that "pretty" container of household detergent. Cooks use a tainted can of soup. Cars are left running in closed garages. Family members combine too many drugs.

Although many poisons are commonly found in the home, they are not usually concocted into deadly brews. Household goods are often locked up. Food that looks or smells funny is immediately thrown away. Cars are turned off before the garage door closes. Adults take responsibility for the medicines they are taking.

In other words, poisoning happens much less in real life than it does on television or in best-selling mystery novels. However, poisoning can happen—and when it does, you need to know how to perform first aid care.

Always Contact the Poison Control Center

Put down this book immediately (mark your place, of course!) and find your telephone book. Look up the number of your local poison control center and record it on your list of emergency phone numbers, tape it in your first aid kit, post it on your refrigerator door, and keep it in your glove compartment.

If you suspect someone is suffering from a poison—from food, household detergents, carbon monoxide, or drugs, for example—call that poison control center number first, even before you call an emergency medical team. Why?

When seconds count, you need to know exactly what to do, and that varies depending on what causes the poisoning. Some poisons need to be flushed from the body by way of induced vomiting. Others should never be thrown up because they'll cause more damage to tissues in the body. The poison control center can give you step-by-step instructions of what to do while you're waiting for an ambulance or in the midst of traffic driving to the emergency ward. Be prepared to answer the following questions if possible:

➤ What kind of poison was ingested?

➤ How much and how long ago?

➤ How old is the victim?

➤ What are the symptoms? Has he or she vomited?

➤ Have you given him or her anything to drink? If yes, what?

The more you can tell the poison control center, the more its specialists can help you.

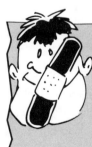

Before You Put the Band-Aid On

Do not follow the instructions on cautionary labels. Household detergents, liquids, and medicines often list instructions that are outdated. Always call your local poison control center instead. The information at the center is cutting edge—much more reliable than a label printed (perhaps) years ago.

When to Induce Vomiting

It sounds logical. To get rid of poison that's been swallowed, the best thing is vomit it up, right? Wrong. In most cases, vomiting is the ideal antidote. But there are times when it is best to keep the poison down and wait for emergency medical help.

Only your local poison control center can tell you for sure whether it's good to vomit. If you cannot reach your local poison control center, you'll have to make a judgment call. Do *not* induce vomiting under any of the following conditions:

➤ Someone has swallowed a cleaning product containing acids or alkalis. They can severely burn throat tissue as he or she throws up.

➤ Someone has swallowed a petroleum-based product. These types of cleaners exude fumes that can cause pneumonia if inhaled. When the poisoned person vomits, these fumes can be inhaled.

➤ The victim is groggy or confused.

➤ He or she is too young to understand and follow directions (such as a baby less than two years old).

➤ You are in doubt. The person's age, the delay time, and the amount ingested all factor into the equation.

> **First Things First**
> If you don't know what the victim has ingested, do *not* induce vomiting. It's far better to be safe than to possibly cause more harm.

How to Induce Vomiting

We can't repeat it enough: call the poison control center immediately when someone eats or drinks a poison. If the authorities at the poison control center give you the green light (excuse the poor choice of colors) to induce vomiting and eliminate the ingested poison, follow these important steps. They tell you exactly how to make someone vomit.

1. Give an adult patient two tablespoons of syrup of ipecac; give a child patient one tablespoon; give a baby (less than 12 months old) two teaspoons.

2. Follow the syrup with four or five glasses of water.

3. Make sure the person's head is lowered to prevent choking. Inside, an adult or child can lie across a bed with his head off the side; outside, he can kneel with his head bent. If a baby swallows poison, keep the baby on your lap with her head down.

4. Try to have the ill person vomit into a bowl so that you can take it to the emergency ward for analysis.

5. If the patient does not vomit, try to induce vomiting again in 20 minutes.

6. If the ill person still does not vomit, don't give him or her any more syrup. Instead, insert your finger in his or her throat to stimulate vomiting via the gagging reflex.

7. After the person vomits, mix one ounce of activated charcoal (if available) in water and have the person sip it. This calms the stomach and acts as a temporary neutralizing antidote.

8. Keep the poisoned person warm.

9. Keep the poisoned person calm. He or she might become panicked. Soothe as best you can. As a last resort, restrain the person using a belt—but only if his or her agitation is so great that it could cause more injury.

10. Mind your ABCs of first aid: Make sure that Airways are clear, Breathing is fairly normal, and Circulation (via pulse) is okay (see Chapter 1)

11. Treat for shock or resuscitate if necessary (see Chapter 3).

12. If the ill person begins to have a convulsion, provide convulsion first aid immediately (see Chapter 25).

First Aid for Poisoning When Vomiting Isn't Advised

Preventing a person from vomiting can be as difficult as inducing him to vomit—especially if he has ingested something particularly nauseating and painful. If you are treating a person who has ingested a poison for which induced vomiting is not advised, follow these steps:

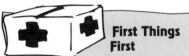

First Things First

If vomiting seems inevitable, turn the person's head to the side so the airways aren't blocked. Try to get him or her to swallow and take deep breaths between vomiting.

1. Call 911 and get medical help as fast as you can.

2. Place the person in a prone position. This will keep the reflex action subdued.

3. Keep the person's head down on the pillow.

4. Keep the person calm and comfortable until help arrives.

Knowing What to Avoid

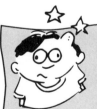

Ouch!

Even if a plant, a chemical, or a medication smells or tastes bad, that doesn't mean it will stop fearless young "explorers." Many children will sample a poison even as they're turning up their noses. So keep all poisons in childproof cabinets or containers and keep them out of sight.

Why does someone eat rhubarb leaves or azalea bushes? Good question—unless you happen to be two years old. Curiosity killed the cat, and it has often harmed a child. Pretty berries or leaves or flowers are easy prey for the young curious mind. Of course, adults might also eat poisonous plants—more likely without realizing it. For example, if you were cooking with rhubarb or eggplant for the first time and you didn't know that the leaves were poisonous, you could be in trouble.

Chemicals are another matter altogether. Sometimes children drink household poisons because the colors on the container are "pretty." (Which is an important reason to childproof your home!) And, unfortunately, there have been cases in which adults swallow household poisons as a means of attempting suicide.

To prevent and deal with any of these scenarios, you should be aware of the types of poisons described in the following tables. Both plant poisons, listed in Table 23.1, and household chemicals, listed in Table 23.2, can be deadly.

Table 23.1   You Are What You Eat: Poisonous Side Dishes to Avoid

Apple seeds	Iris flowers	Poinsettia leaves
Azalea bushes	Jonquil bulbs	Potato greens
Castor bean seeds	Lilies of the Valley	Rhododendron bushes
Daffodil bulbs	Mistletoe berries	Rhubarb leaves
Eggplant leaves	Narcissus bulbs	Sweet Pea seeds
Holly berries	Philodendron leaves	Tomato foliage

Table 23.2   You Are What You Clean: Common Household Poisons

Chemicals in Cleaners

Ammonium Hydroxide	Hydrochloric Acid	Sodium Perborate
Chlorinated Lime	Petroleum solvents	Trisodium Phosphate

Chemicals in Deodorizers

Formaldehyde	Isopropyl Alcohol	Triethylene Glycol

Chemicals in Detergents and Laundry Bleaches

Bichloride of mercury	Potassium Chlorate	Sodium salts
Oxalic acid	Sodium Hypochlorite	Sulfonates

Chemicals in Medicine Cabinets

Antihistamines	Iron tablets	Silver Nitrate
Aspirin	Methyl Salicylate	Tincture of Iodine
Bromides	Multivitamins with iron	Tylenol
Cathartics		

Chemicals in Fuels

Carbon Dioxide	Gasoline Lighter fluid	Natural Gas
Carbon Monoxide	Kerosene Sewer gases	

Ignorance is *not* bliss. Read over this list and learn from it. Keep these items away from children. Please note, however, that these tables are not all-inclusive. They are meant to provide a guide you can use to become more aware of some of the dangers lurking in the average person's kitchen, basement, and backyard. Your local poison center should have a more complete listing.

Drug Overdoses: Accidents Waiting to Happen to Children

Many drug overdoses are accidents involving children who go where they should not tread: the medicine cabinet. When left unsupervised, children can get into pills and medications that can be harmful to their health. Ninety percent of all reported drug poisonings occur in children under five years old.

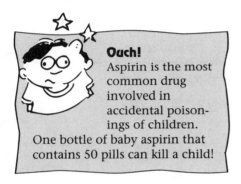

Ouch!
Aspirin is the most common drug involved in accidental poisonings of children. One bottle of baby aspirin that contains 50 pills can kill a child!

Accidental drug overdose poisonings aren't limited to children. An adult might not realize, for example, that she is allergic to a certain medication. Or she might not know what a lethal combination two different types of medication are. Or maybe she just forgets that she already took her prescribed dosage and she takes it again.

Of course, drug overdoses can also be deliberate—and these are the saddest cases of all. More people, especially women, commit suicide by swallowing pills than by any other method. Adolescents also choose pills as the suicide of choice. And even more frightening is the rebellious teen who takes drugs behind his or her parents' backs. They might not consciously want to kill themselves, but teens appear in hospital emergency rooms as "O.D." cases much too often.

The best first aid treatment for accidental or deliberate drug overdose is *prevention*. Follow these safety guidelines:

➤ Childproof all cabinets you keep medicine in, and keep safety caps on all pill bottles.

➤ Clearly label all drugs with universal poison symbols like the ones shown next. Even most adults will remember that they've recently taken the medicine with the skull and crossbones on it and that they should wait a few hours for another dose.

➤ Read *all* labels on medications before taking them, especially the warning labels pertaining to complications that result from medicine combinations.

➤ Keep medicines (even vitamins) away from food. They belong in the medicine cabinet, not the spice drawer.

➤ From time to time, give your children the medicine "rap": Pills are not candy. Medicine is not good to eat. Pills can be downright dangerous.

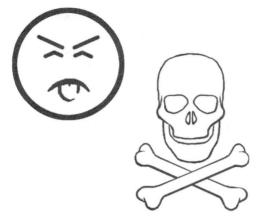

Universal poison symbols: use them to label dangerous drugs and other substances.

Before You Put the Band-Aid On

When kids are on a dangerous "tasting" mission, they often try to hide, especially when they've discovered a fascinating, new (possibly dangerous) object. If you haven't seen your kids in a while, give them a quick once over when they arrive. Do they have stains on their shirts? Do they seem spacey or not themselves? If you suspect something, don't get angry. Just try to determine what your child has been doing. And, at the same time, get ready to go to the emergency ward. It is better to be safe than sorry!

Mushroom Poisoning

In the days of hippies and Carlos Castanada's books about weird mushrooms in South America, mushrooms took on mythical proportions. Today they are what they should be: vegetables to adorn a salad, a sauce, or a main dish. The mushrooms you buy in the supermarket have passed rigid inspection; they are safe to eat. In fact, the majority of mushrooms that grow in the woods are safe to eat.

But there are those few that contain poison, some so deadly that death is almost instantaneous. The best way to avoid eating poison mushrooms? Simple. Do not pick your own mushrooms. Period.

However, accidents do happen, especially when curious children explore the woods on their own.

First Aids
Many people call all poisonous mushrooms *toadstools*. Whatever you call them, it's extremely difficult to tell the "good guys" from the "bad guys." Even experienced, professional woodsmen can have difficulty distinguishing between them.

You'll know something is wrong almost immediately if someone eats poisonous mushrooms. The person will be unable to see clearly, and he or she will act drunk, walking unsteadily, slurring words, and possibly choking. If this happens, call for emergency help immediately. In the interim, follow the steps earlier in this chapter for inducing vomiting.

Poisons That You Don't Eat or Drink

Poison can take many forms. In addition to being swallowed, it can be absorbed through the skin or inhaled. The air you breathe can hold dangerous toxins. And if some chemically strong household products (such as drain cleaners or dishwasher powder) come into contact with your skin, they can cause burns or poisonous reactions almost as bad as if you swallowed them.

How Sweet It Isn't: Breathing in Carbon Monoxide and Other Poisonous Gas

The most common poison gas in the home is carbon monoxide, the odorless, invisible gas that is emitted by cars and some heating systems. Although it is always present, carbon monoxide is only dangerous when it reaches certain levels and when it is trapped in an enclosed space.

Ouch!
Never leave your car running in the garage with the doors closed. Although you might not smell the noxious fumes, they can cause you to quickly lose consciousness—and to die within a few hours.

Symptoms of carbon monoxide poisoning include the following:

Flushed skin

Bright cherry-red lips

Dizziness

Weakness

Headache

Those symptoms ultimately lead to memory loss, confusion, and unconsciousness.

Follow these first-aid steps immediately if someone you love has been overcome by carbon monoxide or some other poisonous gas:

1. If in a garage, turn off the engine and open the doors!

2. Get the victim into fresh air as quickly as possible.

3. Loosen his or her clothing.

4. Call for emergency medical help.

5. Keep the ill person on the ground. Tip the head to the side to ensure clear airways in case he or she vomits.

6. Begin mouth-to-mouth resuscitation, if necessary, while you wait for help to arrive.

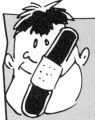

Before You Put the Band-Aid On

Not only are smoke alarms common sights in every house, they are required by law to be working and functioning. The new carbon monoxide alarms look like disc-type smoke alarms, and you can purchase them in any hardware or appliance store. The only problem with these is that, just as super-sensitive smoke alarms can go off when you turn the oven on, carbon monoxide alarms can also go off when the air is perfectly safe. And of course, you can't tell if there really is carbon monoxide in the air the way you can tell that the smoke is just from your oven. Our advice is that you buy a carbon monoxide alarm and have a professional help you decide where to place it to avoid false alarms.

Chemical and Gas Fumes: First Aid Rescue

It can come out of nowhere: a gas burner's pilot light that's left on, a broken heater in the home, a malfunction in your RV's air system, an exterminator's strong fumes, or wet paint left to dry in an unventilated space. When these types of chemical and gas fumes are inhaled or absorbed into the skin, they can be as dangerous as carbon monoxide. And as with carbon monoxide, the first order of first aid business is to get anyone who is affected by such fumes out into the fresh air as soon as possible. To rescue someone in a fume-filled room, follow these steps:

1. Call for help immediately, especially if you are alone. Just in case you too are overcome, it's important to know someone will come along to rescue you. In fact, if the area in question (an underground tank, for example) cannot be ventilated before you enter, you might become a "dead" hero. It's best to wait for professional help to arrive

2. Before you enter the room, take several deep breaths of fresh air. Try to hold your breath as long as you can when you rush into the room.

3. If there is someone else who can help with the rescue attempt, one person can tie a rope around his waist and enter the room while the

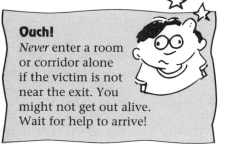

Ouch!
Never enter a room or corridor alone if the victim is not near the exit. You might not get out alive. Wait for help to arrive!

other one waits at the exit, holding the other end of the rope. That way, you can use the rope as a lifeline if the rescuer in the room becomes overcome by fumes.

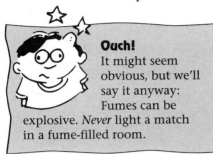

Ouch!
It might seem obvious, but we'll say it anyway: Fumes can be explosive. *Never* light a match in a fume-filled room.

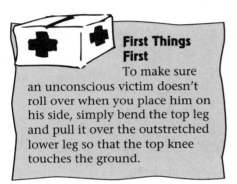

First Things First
To make sure an unconscious victim doesn't roll over when you place him on his side, simply bend the top leg and pull it over the outstretched lower leg so that the top knee touches the ground.

4. If the fumes are visible and circling near the floor, keep your head high. If the fumes appear to be closer to the ceiling, crouch down and walk underneath them.

5. Grasp the overcome person and get him out of the room as fast as you can.

6. Once you're in the fresh air, check the victim's breathing. If he is not breathing, immediately proceed with mouth-to-mouth resuscitation (see Chapter 3), or if you are trained, begin CPR.

If the victim is having trouble breathing, lie him on his back with his head resting on an elevated pillow while you wait for help. (If he is overcome by smoke, see Chapter 26, "Smoke Inhalation.")

If the victim is unconscious, position him on his side to keep airways clear in case vomiting occurs. Place a pillow under his head as shown in the following illustration.

If the victim seems to be clear-headed, awake, and breathing fine, have him lie on his back. Elevate his legs by placing a pillow under the lower legs; this keeps blood circulating and ensures that the brain gets plenty of oxygen.

Position an unconscious victim on his side and bend the top knee so that he won't roll over.

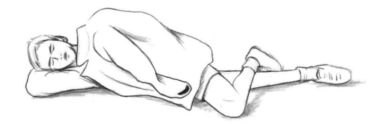

7. Check the victim's skin and eyes for possible contamination. If eyes are very irritated or burned, it's possible that they've come in contact with chemical fumes. Flush the eyes immediately with cool water. (Chapter 11 covers first aid treatment for eye injuries.)

8. If the skin is burned from fumes or from contact with chemicals, pour cool water on the wound and try to flush out the poison. (Chapter 19 covers first aid treatment for skin irritations.)

9. Even if the victim seems fine once you've rescued him or her, it's a good idea to make a doctor's appointment within the next few days. Inhalation of poisonous fumes can cause side effects such as nerve damage, respiratory problems, memory loss, and muscle aches, some of which don't appear right away.

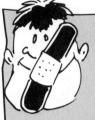

Before You Put the Band-Aid On

Sometimes the effects of chemical and poisonous fumes are cumulative; they go unnoticed for months or even years. Recent studies have found that the solvents used in dry cleaning can possibly cause certain cancers, respiratory ailments, or sterility. Although those studies are not conclusive, it's wise to take the following precautions:

➤ Take your dry cleaning out of the plastic bag as soon as you get home. This gives your clothes time to "breathe."

➤ Wear clothes multiple times before you dry clean them.

➤ Try not to buy clothes that cannot be hand or machine-washed.

Drug Overdose: When Prevention Is Too Late

In theworst of all possible scenarios, if your preventative efforts seem to have failed, and your teen, friend, or spouse doesn't respond, you'll need to take him or her to the emergency room—quickly. To make sure you understand what is going on in order to give the professionals there as much information as possible, you'll need to be able to recognize signs of a drug overdose. The top ten signs include:

1. Extremely constricted pupils (pinpoints) or extremely over-dilated pupils

2. Off-kilter gait

3. Excessive chattering that makes no sense

4. Lethargy

5. Rapid and sudden mood swings

6. Inability to focus or concentrate

7. Excessive amount of energy

8. Unwarranted violent anger

9. A "stoned" quality in which the person acts like a robot, somewhere in outer space

10. Paranoia, and in extreme cases, hallucinations

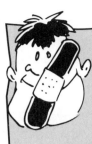

Before You Put the Band-Aid On

It's the parents' worst nightmare for a teenager to be actively using alcohol or other drugs. Some parents deny there is a problem, even if the telltale signs are right in front of them. If you, as a parent, notice any of the following signs in your child, call a support intervention line for help.

Unexplained need for money

Drop in grades

Hanging around with a new group of "wild" peers

Severe depression and isolation

Lack of appetite

Secretive behavior

Fits of screaming anger (directed at you)

If someone exhibits three or more symptoms over a period of a few weeks, seek help—both psychological and physical. Family therapy is especially good for adolescents in trouble.

Treating the Eight Most Common Overdoses

Drug overdose is a serious matter. Unfortunately, many adults and teens suffer from its slings. Usually drug overdose is a mask, hiding other problems: insecurity, self-loathing, a sense of failure, or deep and unabiding depression. These problems must also be addressed in order to prevent the "self-medication" so many drug addicts use from becoming a dangerous overdose. Here are the seven most common drugs that are used for "escape" and that can lead to overdoses. Recognize them and understand them. You could save a life.

Alcohol

We don't often think of liquor as a drug, but it is the most often abused drug of all. Whether excessive drinking results from a genetic problem, an emotional problem, or a combination of the two, there is help. That help might come in the form of Alcoholics Anonymous and other support groups or medication. But sometimes you don't have the luxury of time. Acute intoxication can occur when someone drinks too much in a short period of time; eventually his or her body becomes "toxic" with alcohol, and an overdose occurs. His or her body is literally poisoned by the alcohol.

Blood alcohol levels are used to gauge the amount of alcohol in the blood. If someone's blood alcohol level is high, it means that there is simply too much alcohol in the blood, and it's "crowding out" the life-sustaining fluids necessary for a person to function as an alert, thinking individual. High levels mean that a person should not drive; higher levels can lead to overdose.

Police consider the result of drinking more than two drinks in an hour to be dangerous. But many people can tolerate a great deal more alcohol before being close to an overdose. An alcoholic cannot gauge his or her drunkenness. But you can. You can bet that a person has too high a blood alcohol level if he exhibits a stumbling gait, flushed face and clammy skin, garbled speech, sleepwalking, or erratic mood swings. All are signs that the person has had more than enough—definitely too much to drive home.

How can you tell if someone who has drank alcohol needs medical attention? Call for help if the person's skin is very clammy and cold, if he or she is unconscious, if the pulse is very irregular and faint, or if the breathing becomes labored. If you suspect that someone has overdosed on alcohol, proceed with these steps:

1. Call for help. In the meantime, don't try to reason with him or her because intoxication can make people violent. Instead try to be reassuring.

2. Try to wake the intoxicated person. Acute intoxication can cause people to fall asleep where they lie. It can also cause unconsciousness. If you cannot awaken the person, call for emergency help.

3. Check the person's breathing. If it is irregular, place the person on his or her side to keep airways clear. This also prevents choking in the event of vomiting.

4. Check his or her pulse. If it is weak, rapid, or irregular, call for emergency help. Perform mouth-to-mouth resuscitation if necessary (see Chapter 3).

5. Observe the intoxicated person's skin. If it is clammy, cold, and pale, cover him or her with a loose blanket while you wait for help.

Depressants: Quaaludes, Sedatives, and So On

These are the other "depressants" that actually slow the body down to such an extent that they can kill. For example, Phenobarbital and barbiturates are extremely dangerous, especially when mixed with alcohol. They are not regularly prescribed and are considered "street drugs." Depressants are "downers." Take too many of these and you'll feel even more depressed—and in danger of overdosing. An overdose of depressants brings on unconsciousness, which rapidly becomes a full-fledged coma. If the victim is not rushed to a hospital for a stomach pump, he or she can die.

First Aids
Antidepressants combat a chemical imbalance in the brain that causes clinical depression. When combined with psychotherapy, these medications can prevent self-destructive habits. They stop depression and they prevent overdoses because a person loses the need to "self-medicate" himself.

Hallucinogens Such as LSD and Herbal Ecstasy

Hallucinogens are also street drugs that are not ever prescribed. LSD (or acid), PCP (angel dust), mescaline, ecstasy, and some types of mushrooms can all cause hallucinations and a good or bad "trip." People under the influence of these seem far away. They might talk to invisible people or objects, or they might babble. And if they have a bad trip, they might act paranoid, alternately screaming and acting catatonic. Perception, sensation, thought, emotion, and self-awareness are all skewed.

If someone overdoses on an hallucinogen, she might believe herself to be omnipotent. The person can get physically hurt as she attempts to fly or to walk through fire or do whatever the mind is portraying. If you suspect someone is on a bad trip, follow these steps:

1. Calm the person down. Be reassuring and keep your voice low as you try to keep him or her from physical harm.

2. Try to talk the person "down" from the scary place in his or her mind's eye. Make sure the surroundings are safe and familiar.

3. Take the person to a hospital. If you can get someone to help you, all the better. Two people are better than one in emergencies. If the victim is violent, resists help, or attacks you, call 911 immediately.

Inhalants Such as Glue and "White-Out"

Unfortunately, teenagers today are trying a new kind of high: chemical inhalants such as airplane glue, paint, kerosene, gas, nail polish, and lighter fluid. Although they might get high, they also get sick. Earlier in this chapter, you learned about the dangers of inhaled chemical fumes. If you find someone to be ill from "inhaling" (also called "huffing" or "sniffing"), follow this course of treatment:

1. Call for emergency medical help immediately.

2. Remove the inhalant and any accompanying apparatus (such as cotton balls, straws, or soaked paper bags) from the area of the person's mouth and nose.

3. Check breathing. If necessary, perform mouth-to-mouth resuscitation (or CPR if you are trained to do so).

4. Open windows to increase ventilation of fresh air.

5. If the person is unconscious, cover him or her with a loose blanket and treat for shock as you learned in Chapter 3.

Not a New Dance

Autoasphyxiation has been around for a while, picked up by teens as they become interested in sex. It involves choking or strangling yourself or a friend with a cord or a rope to the point of near unconsciousness. It is used in sex acts and in masturbation, particularly among teenage boys. The resulting "high" comes from the adrenaline rush combined with decreased delivery of oxygen to the brain. Because the rope is usually hung from, say, a shower stall or a light fixture, several teenagers have died by accidentally going too far. They fainted or were strangled when they couldn't release the knot.

Signs of autoasphyxiation use include bruises and red marks around the neck. As a parent, you might also watch out for ropes and other unusual equipment in a teen's room, an unusual amount of time spent in the bathroom, and withdrawal from family and friends.

First aid treatment for this is difficult unless you catch the person in the act. He or she must be taken down from the hanging position immediately and taken to the emergency ward. But, because this practice is usually performed when parents aren't home, you might not know about it until it is too late. Therefore, the best first aid is prevention. If you have any reason to suspect that your child is playing around with this, contact an intervention hotline or seek a therapist. Your teen will need help before it is too late.

Stimulants: Amphetamines, Cocaine, and So On

As the word implies, stimulants are drugs that act as direct opposites of depressants. They stimulate the mind—at least initially—and ward off sleepiness. They are also highly addictive and have ruined the lives of many people who have started snorting or popping them. The most common stimulants are amphetamines, "speed," crack, "CAT" (crystal methamphetamine), and cocaine.

Early signs of stimulant use include overconfidence, extreme energy, euphoria, and excessive talking. After only a few days, addiction sets in. The symptoms include:

Confusion and paranoia	Delusion
Violent and aggressive behavior	Anxiety attacks that mimic heart attacks
Antisocial actions	

Because of stimulants' addictive nature, over time a person needs more and more of the drug to get high. As a result, stimulant overdoses are seen quite often in the emergency room.

Follow these steps if you think someone has overdosed on cocaine or another stimulant:

1. Immediately call for emergency help.

2. Try to prevent the person from hurting him or herself.

3. Be calm and reassuring. Talk in a low voice.

4. If the person is lying down and is shaking or unconscious, turn him or her to the side to keep airways clear and to prevent him or her from choking on vomit.

5. Loosen clothing.

6. Loosely place a warm blanket over the person.

Tranquilizers Such as Valium, Halycon, and Librium

There was a time when doctors prescribed Valium for almost everything. Tranquilizers are still used to help people who suffer from panic attacks, anxiety, and insomnia. Unfortunately, they can become addictive and must be carefully monitored. Tranquilizers are considered a controlled substance, and prescriptions can only be filled a certain number of times each year. If someone overdoses on tranquilizers, he or she will fall asleep and will eventually become unconscious. Follow these steps if you suspect a tranquilizer overdose:

1. Call for help immediately. The person's stomach must be pumped.

2. Try to keep the victim up and moving around. Do everything you can to prevent him or her from falling asleep before help arrives.

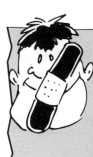

Before You Put the Band-Aid On

Sometimes drug withdrawal can mimic drug overdose. If someone has abruptly stopped taking medication or has stopped drinking, it is possible that he or she will exhibit the same signs as with an overdose (rapid pulse, disorientation, clammy skin, and more). If these symptoms occur, take the person to a hospital to ensure that he or she receives the right type of care.

Narcotics Such as Heroin and Opium

These are the most deadly drugs of all. Highly addictive and highly dangerous to the body, narcotics include opium and its derivatives, morphine and codeine, heroin, Demerol, and methadone. Because narcotics are not regulated, it's difficult to inject a safe amount, and overdoses happen frequently. Symptoms of a narcotics overdose include:

Lethargy	Contracted pupils (to pinpoints)
Profuse sweating	Clammy skin
Low temperature	Muscle relaxation
Weak pulse	Weak breathing
Sleep, leading to a coma	

To treat an overdose of narcotics, follow these steps:

1. Call for help immediately.

2. Try to rouse the person who has overdosed, slapping his cheek gently if necessary.

3. If the victim is lying down, turn him to the side to keep airways clear and to prevent choking if he begins to vomit.

4. Don't show your anger or dismay—at least right now. Instead, reassure the victim as you wait for help to arrive.

The Least You Need to Know

➤ Always call your local poison control center before administering first aid for poisoning. Keep the number handy.

➤ Sometimes vomiting up a poison is the right thing to do, but when the poison is lye or a petroleum-based household products, vomiting can burn the throat.

➤ Carbon monoxide is an odorless, invisible, and very poisonous gas. Never leave a car running in a closed garage, and have your gas furnace checked yearly for leaks.

➤ If you have to rescue someone from an enclosed room full of chemical fumes, call for help first. If anything happens to you, help will be on its way for both of you.

➤ Aspirin is the major cause of accidental drug overdose in children. Keep all medicine in a childproof cabinet!

➤ Drug overdose always requires a visit to the emergency room; get the victim there as quickly as possible.

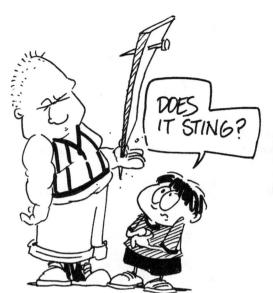

Puncture Wounds and Splinters

One of the jobs of being a parent is to take splinters out. And it's not easy to see a child's eyes, tearful and red, as she holds out a finger with the slightest edge of dark wood sticking out—wood from the toy cabinet, from the attic floor, from the piano stool.

Splinters and puncture wounds are very similar: a foreign object punctures or "impales" the skin. The difference between the two is a matter of degree. Splinters are relatively minor, and you can usually handle their removal without outside help. Puncture wounds, on the other hand, penetrate further below the skin, possibly damaging blood vessels, muscles, and nerves. For them, you'll always need emergency help.

The operative words here are sterilize, remove, clean, and bandage. But within these elements lies a whole world of procedure.

A Splinter Is a Splinter Is a Splinter...

Who hasn't had a splinter at one time or another in their lives? A tiny sliver of glass, a minuscule piece of wood, a slender slice of plastic or metal slides right under the skin and lodges there to cause pain. These splinters might hurt, but if they are removed properly, there will be no infection.

A person knows he or she has a splinter because of the pain at the penetration site. There also might be some swelling and redness. To take out a splinter, follow these step-by-step instructions:

1. Place the instrument you'll be using to take out the splinter nearby. This is usually a plain sewing needle or a tweezers, or both.

2. Wash your hands thoroughly with soap and water to make conditions as sterile as possible. Also wash the splinter site.

3. Sterilize the sewing needle and tweezers you will use to take out the splinter by either dropping them in boiling water for ten minutes or heating them over the flame of a match or lighter. (Wipe off any black carbon deposits with a sterile gauze pad.)

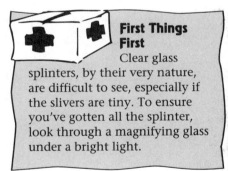

First Things First
Clear glass splinters, by their very nature, are difficult to see, especially if the slivers are tiny. To ensure you've gotten all the splinter, look through a magnifying glass under a bright light.

4. Using the sewing needle or tweezers, gently and carefully brush away the skin around the splinter, layer by layer.

5. When enough of the splinter is exposed to be able to grab it, use your tweezers and pull it out. If the splinter is small, continue to use the sewing needle, pushing out the splinter from the skin.

6. Brush the skin with the sewing needle a little more to make sure you've gotten all of the splinter. Think of the needles as a little broom, pushing away the skin tissue surrounding the point of insertion. This is especially important when a sliver of glass is the culprit.

7. Wash the wound area with water, whether it's bleeding or not. Apply an antibacterial ointment.

8. Cover the clean wound site with a Band-Aid or gauze pad and tape.

Puncture Wounds

A puncture wound leaves a small hole on the surface of the skin, but below the surface the foreign object is deeply embedded. The wound's initial contact diffuses under the skin, spreading out its destruction to cause bleeding and tissue damage.

Most puncture wounds are caused by objects bigger than splinters. Arrows, large shards of metal and glass, nails, even sharp sticks of wood, can puncture the skin and damage underlying tissue.

The Hidden Problems with Punctures

Any puncture wound is prone to infection because of the depth of the foreign object's invasion. Punctures particularly vulnerable are those in which a foreign object:

➤ Goes through clothing, taking particles of cloth with it as it enters the skin

➤ Breaks up into smaller pieces as it becomes embedded under the skin

➤ Is extremely dirty, such as a puncture caused by a rusty nail

➤ Enters the body through the foot, which can "push" the object in further as a person tries to limp toward help

First Things First
Signs of infection include redness at the puncture site, swelling (especially if blood vessels have been damaged), tenderness near the wound, and pain at site. You are not out of the woods if these signs do not appear within the day of the injury. Oozing pus can appear at the site days after the accident.

Yes, it's true that puncture wounds are more likely to be infected. But that doesn't mean you have to immediately rush the victim to the emergency ward to be checked. What it does mean is that you need to keep an eye on the wound. Watch the wound for several days to see if it is healing. It also means changing the dressing frequently, keeping the wound clean, and applying new applications of antiseptic.

If after a few days, the wound scabs over, the redness disappears, and swelling at the site of impact goes down, you can usually say that the danger of infection is gone. If, however, pus continues (or starts) to drain from the site and the redness persists, it could very well mean that infection has set in—or that the foreign object left a souvenir. (This is particularly dangerous because even very small foreign objects that are deeply embedded in the skin can cause infection and blood poisoning.) We suggest taking the victim to the physician, a medicenter, or the emergency ward for better treatment. An antibiotic might have to be prescribed to fight the infection.

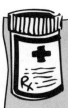

First Aids

Tetanus is an infectious, sometimes fatal disease, caused by a bacterium that invades the body through wounds. Its symptoms include violent spasms and paralysis of the neck and jaw. For this reason, the disease is often called "lockjaw."

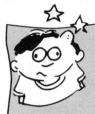

Ouch!

If the person with the puncture wound has not had a tetanus shot within ten years, it's a good idea to get a booster. Tetanus bacteria thrives in dark, deep places with little air—just the environment created by a puncture wound.

Sometimes when a puncture wound occurs, the object does not remain embedded in the tissue. This is what happens when a person steps on a rusty nail or leans against a sharp edge. In this case, treatment should still include cleaning the wound and applying an antiseptic, but we strongly urge you to see a physician. The victim might need a tetanus shot. The rusty nail could cause a bad infection or tetanus if you do not take care of the situation.

Treating a Puncture Wound

The first rule to remember is do not try to take out an object embedded in a puncture wound by yourself. Any movement can cause more tissue damage or more bleeding. Call for emergency help and keep the puncture site immobile using these steps:

1. Gently clean the wound with soap and water, and then cover the wound with a loose gauze pad and adhesive tape.

2. Poke a hole in the bottom of an paper cup wide enough to slip over the exposed end of the foreign object.

3. Gently tape the cup in place. (Make a "fence" of cardboard or newspaper if you don't have a cup.)

4. If the puncture wound is on the arm, further immobilize the wound by keeping the arm tight against the torso. Do this by winding a scarf or belt around both the arm (further down from the wound) and lower torso.

If the puncture wound is on the leg, wind the cloth or belt around both legs, adding a sturdy piece of wood to the back of the legs for extra insurance.

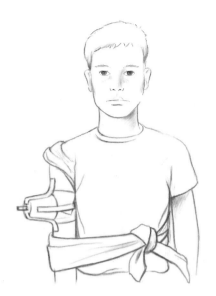

Immobilize a puncture wound to prevent it from causing more damage.

Before You Put the Band-Aid On

One of the reasons first aid kits were invented was so that a person could have a handy, compact kit for emergency medicine if he was far from civilization. Hopefully, if you suffer a puncture wound when you're in, say, the deep forest, you'll have your handy kit with you. If not, do the best you can. Necessity is the mother of invention, after all. You can use a piece of shirt instead of a gauze pad, keep it in place with a belt, and use spring water to clean a wound. Do whatever you have to do until you can find your way to a phone or a hospital.

Dealing with Bleeding

As with any bleeding wound, applying direct pressure stops the flow of blood. (See Chapter 3 for more information on bleeding.) If the injured person is bleeding profusely, do not immediately immobilize the wound. Before you take any other action, stop the bleeding using these steps:

1. Cut any clothing away from the wound.

2. Wash your hands thoroughly to avoid further infection to the wound.

3. Put a sterile gauze pad *around* the embedded object, but not directly on it. If the object is protruding, place the gauze pad on the skin and encircle the site of penetration. (Remember the earlier instructions for treating puncture wounds. Cover any protruding objects with a paper cup, cutting a slit in the middle of it so that the rim will touch the skin. This will keep infection at bay until you can get help.)

233

4. Press firmly on the gauze pad.

5. Keep the wound elevated above heart level, if possible, to lessen the blood flow to the site.

Before You Put the Band-Aid On

There are many old myths that abound, but some of them aren't myths at all. One of these has to do with bleeding puncture wounds. Of course, if bleeding is copious, the flow must be squelched. But a little blood is not necessarily a bad thing. Blood, like any other fluid, washes away contaminants as it seeps out of the skin. It's best not to let the blood seep out for any length of time (infection can still set in!), and it won't really help to squeeze the wound site to get more blood out. (This will only help imbed the object more.) But a little blood means that possible infections might be washed out.

The Least You Need to Know

➤ Splinters and puncture wounds are different from cuts and open bruises. Here, a foreign object becomes embedded in the flesh, and it must be removed before infection sets in.

➤ Splinters are usually minor problems and easily can be removed with a sterilized sewing needle and tweezers.

➤ Puncture wounds involve larger shards of glass, wood, or metal that become embedded in tissue below the surface of the skin. First aid for puncture wounds always requires medical attention. Never try to remove the object that has punctured the skin. Keep the area immobile until help arrives.

➤ Signs of infection include redness, pain, swelling, and tenderness at the wound site.

➤ Get a tetanus shot!

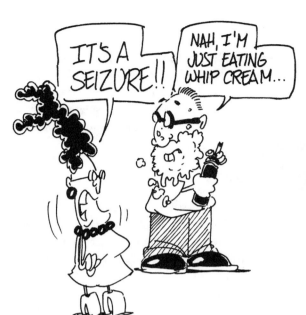

Chapter 25

Seizures and Convulsions

In This Chapter

➤ Signs of a seizure

➤ Steps to take when someone has a seizure

➤ When a seizure or convulsion can be dangerous

➤ What to do when a child under six has a seizure

Whether you call it a seizure or a convulsion, the condition is the same—and it can appear terrifying to someone who doesn't know what's going on. Although it might look like the person having a seizure is in terrible trouble and awful pain, most seizures are not dangerous at all. You merely have to let them run their course.

The danger of seizures comes from the root of the episode, not the actual convulsions. A seizure can be the result of a brain tumor, brain damage, measles, meningitis, or even lead poisoning. On the other hand, a seizure can have a harmless root. It can be genetically transferred from parent to child and be nothing more than a momentary electrical "blitz" within the passageways of the brain. However, studies have shown that continuous recurrent convulsions can affect short-term memory.

The moral of this story? If someone you are with has a seizure, get him or her to a hospital. There is no immediate danger, but the surrounding facts need to be examined.

A Seizure's Symptoms

A seizure or convulsion happens suddenly. There's rarely any signal. Nor can the person about to have a seizure say, "Watch out! Here comes a seizure!" The person hasn't a clue that a seizure is about to occur—unless he or she has had them in the past. Symptoms can be dramatic and scary to behold (which is usually what's called a *grand mal* seizure), or they can be so mild that the few seconds of lost consciousness goes by without anyone being aware of it (which is called an *absence* or a *petit mal* seizure).

Seizures Come in Many Sizes and Shapes

There are more than 20 types of seizures, which are distinguished by determining where the electrical signaling in the brain misfired and how far the "brainstorm" spreads. If the misfiring occurs in the area of the brain that governs the movement of a particular limb, only that limb will jerk spasmodically. If the misfiring occurs in the area of the brain that controls vision or hearing, a person might suffer from hallucinations. And if the misfiring occurs in the limbic system, which covers the emotional arena, a person might become hysterical and anxious. (See Chapter 16 on the brain.) These singularly symptomatic seizures are called "partial" or "focal" seizures.

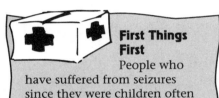

First Things First

People who have suffered from seizures since they were children often get warning signs of an upcoming episode. Sometimes they will feel "butterflies" in their stomachs. Sometimes they hear music or a loud roaring. And sometimes they smell a distinct odor before they "black out" and the seizure begins.

Usually, people know they have seizures; it's a condition many people have had to deal with since birth. Those people usually wear Medic Alert bracelets or necklaces to alert others of their condition, and they usually carry appropriate anti-epileptic medication (such as Klonopin or Dilantin). These people know what to do and what to expect. There is no need to take one of them to an emergency ward when he suffers a seizure.

The symptoms of a grand mal or partial seizure can include the following:

A sudden loss of consciousness combined with a fall to the ground

Rigid body stance, followed by uncontrollable spasms, jerking, or twitching

Eyes rolled upward

Face and lips turn blue

Foaming at the mouth or drooling

Loss of bladder or bowel control

Biting of the tongue

Temporary breathing stoppage

A seizure can last as long as 90 seconds.

Why Seizures?

There are many reasons why people have convulsions or seizures. Epilepsy is the most common, but there are other causes:

High fever

Head injury

Alcohol withdrawal

Drug use or withdrawal

Brain tumors

Poison

Electric shock

Hyperventilation

Shock (because not enough oxygen is being sent to the brain)

Hypotension (which is very low blood pressure)

Hypoxia (a decrease of oxygen in the arteries)

Hypoglycemia (low blood sugar), especially in a diabetic

First Aids

Epilepsy is a disorder of the nervous system that starts with a burst of abnormal electrical activity within the passageways of the brain. This misfiring causes a "glitz" in the normal brain function, which is outwardly displayed as a convulsion or seizure that occurs again and again over time. The hallmark of epilepsy is the quick way in which a seizure takes place. A flickering light or a lack of sleep can trigger a seizure.

The Dangers of Seizures

As we have pointed out, seizures by themselves are not necessarily dangerous except when they occur for the first time in an otherwise healthy individual. But because of the possibility that an underlying medical condition has caused the convulsion, it's important to get the person to the emergency ward for help as soon as the seizure has passed.

The other danger of seizure is purely environmental. A person can have a seizure and fall to a hard floor, injuring his or her head. A person can have a seizure while swimming, and he or she will be in danger of drowning. A person can have a convulsion while driving, which brings up a lot of serious side effects. And, if a seizure lasts longer than five minutes, there is always the possibility of heart, kidney, or brain damage.

Because of the potential dangers in these situations, people should be aware of each other's medical history, especially when traveling on business or pleasure. Medication storage should be noted, and everyone should know what to do for first aid care if a person in the group has a seizure.

Waiting for the Seizure to Subside: The "DON'Ts" of First Aid

There's very little you can do while someone is having a seizure except to move any furniture out of harm's way. You can loosen the person's clothing and try to help him to the ground as he starts to fall.

However, there are a lot of things you should NOT do when a seizure is taking place. These "do nots" are critical.

DO NOT...

➤ Attempt to restrain the person having the seizure. You can cause the person to tear muscles or break a bone.

➤ Force anything between the person's teeth. This can result in broken teeth—or a broken finger—yours.

➤ Throw ice cold water on the person in the hopes it will "shake" him or her out of it. Not only will splashing water have no effect, but it can cause the person to choke!

Before You Put the Band-Aid On

It's often said that placing a pencil or tongue depressor between the teeth of a person having a seizure helps prevent him or her from biting off the tongue.

Wrong. Although it's almost been *de rigueur* in health education (and movies about Alexander the Great and Caesar of Rome), this technique does nothing. The worst that can happen is that a person will bite his or her tongue and it will bleed. If you place something else in the person's mouth like a pencil or tongue depressor, he or she may break it and swallow part of it.

After the Fall: Treatment When the Seizure Is Over

After the victim comes out of a convulsion, there are some first aid steps to take to ensure comfort and safety:

1. Call for emergency help. If possible, try not to leave the victim's side (in case there are any complications).

2. Check for any medic alert bracelets or neck tags, if the person is not a family member or close friend. It is possible the person is an epileptic or has another condition that requires specific medical attention. Be ready to tell the emergency team when they arrive.

3. Check the victim's breathing. If he or she is still not breathing, or breathing with difficulty, perform mouth-to-mouth resuscitation. (See Chapter 3 for more information.)

4. As the person comes out of the seizure, do not startle him or her. Do not act panicky or ask any questions. Let him or her rest. After a seizure, a person might be confused, very sleepy, or even combative and violent. Don't be alarmed. It's a normal part of "coming out" of a seizure.

5. Turn the person's head (or his or her entire body) to the side to prevent choking if he or she vomits.

6. Observe whether there are any burns around the victim's mouth. If there are, it's possible the convulsions were due to poisoning.

7. The person who suffered the seizure might fall into a deep sleep at this point. He or she might snore quite loudly. It's quite common and nothing to be alarmed about.

Seizures in Children

Although seizures in children are the most frightening of all, they, too, are relatively harmless after the convulsions have passed. In childhood, the first signs of epilepsy might appear. Further, high fever or severe gastrointestinal upsets can cause convulsions. Seizures can also become a permanent or temporary aftereffect of rheumatic fever.

However, it's important to seek medical care immediately if this is the first seizure you've seen. It can be a symptom of something serious, and medication might be needed.

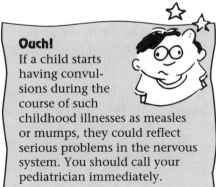

Ouch!
If a child starts having convulsions during the course of such childhood illnesses as measles or mumps, they could reflect serious problems in the nervous system. You should call your pediatrician immediately.

If a child is having a seizure, you should follow the same first aid procedures as with an adult—with one exception. If the seizure is the result of high fever, follow these first aid steps instead of the earlier ones:

1. Give your child baby ibuprofen or acetaminophen after the seizure has passed. (Avoid aspirin because of the risk of Reye's syndrome; see Chapter 13.)

2. Sponge him or her off with lukewarm water. (Warm water is more soothing than cold.)

3. Never place your child in the tub. If your child has another seizure, he or she could drown!

These three measures should lower your child's temperature without causing dangerous side effects. By lowering the temperature, you decrease the chances of another seizure.

The Least You Need to Know

➤ Whether you call it a seizure or a convulsion the condition looks much worse than it is. However, you should always seek medical attention after a seizure because there could be a serious medical condition that caused it.

➤ Never put anything between the teeth of someone having a seizure.

➤ While the seizure is taking place, you should try to catch the victim before he or she falls, loosen clothing, move furniture or other objects out of the way, and wait. That's all.

➤ After the seizure subsides, be calm. Let the victim rest, and give first aid if the person vomits or stops breathing.

➤ If seizures last more than 90 seconds or occur in succession, it can signal a serious medical condition. It can also cause liver, kidney, or brain damage. Get medical help promptly!

➤ Children usually have seizures as a result of high fever. Call your pediatrician, and treat with ibuprofen or acetaminophen and a lukewarm sponge bath.

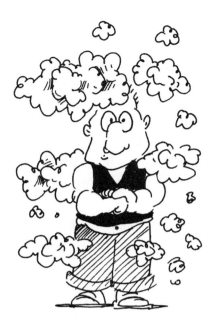

Smoke Inhalation

We all inhale smoke of some sort or another every day. Air pollution, smog, second-hand (or first-hand!) cigarette smoke—all of these things draw smoke into our lungs with every breath.

But there is good news. The respiratory system has wonderful protective devices to keep lungs clear of smoke. In this chapter, you will learn how the respiratory system works to filter impurities and provide life-sustaining oxygen. You will also learn how this selfsame system can become "overloaded," creating a potentially life-threatening situation: smoke inhalation.

And most important, you will learn what to do if you suddenly find yourself or someone else in a burning house with no air to breathe, or in a room (perhaps a kitchen) where smoke is accumulating with no way out.

Smoke Gets in Your Lungs

When you breathe in a gulp of air, it travels down your windpipe (or trachea). Rings of cartilage keep the windpipe from collapsing so that the air can easily move through the windpipe, past your collarbone, your ribs, and to the center of your chest.

There, your windpipe divides into two tubes called the bronchial tubes, each of which leads to one of your lungs. By the time your gulp of air reaches the lungs, most dirt particles, smog, dust, and bacteria have already been swept away by the hairs in your nose, by a strong sneeze, or a sudden cough.

But just in case that's not enough, the lungs themselves have protective devices to keep poisons such as smoke, dust, and other the everyday pollutants at bay.

The bronchial tubes break down into millions of tiny tubes, called bronchioles. Within these bronchioles are little pockets called alveoli (which almost rhymes with ravioli). These alveoli (the plural of the singular alveolus), which are surrounded by capillaries, are only a membrane away from the blood cells that are clambering for the oxygen "food" you've just inhaled. The alveoli are the moat around the castle—the fortress wall that keeps enemies at bay.

The components of the lungs.

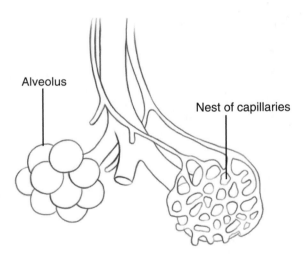

Alveolus

Nest of capillaries

Because it's important that the oxygen not be tainted, the human's genetic makeup contains a kind of vacuum cleaner to catch wayward dust. The alveoli are covered with wet and sticky mucous. Dust particles (which have also broken down into minute cells) stick to these mucous walls.

Now comes the cleaning-up part. The alveoli also contain mucous cells with membrane "arms" called cilia. Cilia resemble sweeping, swaying tentacles. The dust catches on the cilia and is swayed back, out of the lung, into the part of the throat (the esophagus) that leads to the stomach. Acids in the stomach area begin to make short shrift of the "poison." Your body cells receive the clean oxygen and eliminate carbon dioxide waste that is exhaled out of your lungs.

Unfortunately, when you become overcome with smoke, this process of "cleaning," receiving, and eliminating breaks down. There are just too many foreign particles for the cilia to sweep them all away. Even the automatic "defense mechanisms" of sneezing and coughing will not help clear your lungs of smoke. They are merely a drop in the bucket.

When you suffer from smoke inhalation, your body does not get the oxygen it needs to do its job—and the lungs can become damaged as well.

If There's Smoke, Does There Have to Be Fire?

Obviously, smoke is a by-product of fire, but you don't have to be locked up in an unventilated burning room to be overcome by smoke. Smoke inhalation also can occur from minor fires, such as:

➤ Fireplaces with faulty air ducts

➤ Stovetop fires

➤ The smoldering at the onset of electrical fires

➤ Broiler fires

➤ Grill fires in improperly ventilated porches and decks

➤ Smoldering furniture or mattresses (courtesy of sloppy and dangerous smokers who do not put out their matches or cigarettes)

Smoke Signals

The signs of smoke inhalation vary. Minor problems include irritated eyes, coughing jags, and general weakness—which can turn into more serious symptoms if the victim does not get away from the smoke.

To treat smoke inhalation follow these steps:

1. The first order of business is to get the victim into the fresh air!

2. Have the victim sit down until he or she begins to feel better.

3. After coughing has subsided, offer a glass of water to calm a burning throat.

4. Place a cool washcloth over the victim's eyes and forehead.

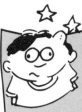

Ouch!
Although minor incidents are not medical emergencies, they can turn into emergencies if the person involved has asthma, allergic bronchitis, emphysema, or any other chronic pulmonary disease. These people are more sensitive to smoke, and what is minor in a normal person can wreak havoc in a sensitive one. Even smoke from an ordinary campfire can cause a severe asthma attack! A good rule of thumb is to seek medical attention for any asthmatic who is wheezing, no matter how minor the inhalation seems. This especially holds true for young children!

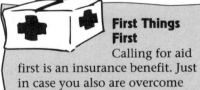

First Things First
Calling for aid first is an insurance benefit. Just in case you also are overcome with smoke, someone will be on the way to help.

Minor incidents do not usually require special medical care. Trust your instincts and your methods of observation. If the person seems fine and does not have a lingering cough, he or she will not need immediate medical attention. But it is always a good idea to call the family physician and have him or her give the "all clear."

Symptoms of serious smoke inhalation requiring first aid include:

Continued wheezing and coughing

An inability to breathe

Choking

Lightheadedness

Ash, black char, or smoke around the mouth and nose

Weakness and lethargy that could lead to unconsciousness

To treat a serious case of smoke inhalation, in which the victim is suffering from the symptoms described above, follow these steps:

1. Call for help.

2. Drag the injured person away from the smoke—without injuring yourself.

3. Check the victim's breathing. If he or she is having difficulty, perform mouth-to-mouth resuscitation (or CPR, if trained) until help arrives. (See Chapter 3 for more information.)

4. Cover the victim with a blanket. If he or she is lying on the cold ground, place a blanket underneath as well.

5. Loosen clothes around the neck and torso to help breathing.

6. To prevent possible shock, make sure the victim is lying on his or her back, with a pillow behind the head if she is having difficulty breathing, or a pillow elevating the legs and feet if all seems well.

7. If the victim is unconscious, turn his or her head to the side to prevent possible vomit from choking him or her.

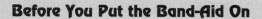

Before You Put the Band-Aid On

Cigarette smoking might not be an immediate first aid problem, but it certainly does a job on your lungs (and other parts of your body). The tar and soot from cigarette smoke is more than the protective cilia can handle. They become paralyzed. The cigarette smoke eventually gets inside the cells and, combined with the mucus manufactured in the alveoli, creates sticky balls that clog passageways and cells. And, oh yes, one more thing: your healthy pink lungs eventually turn black.

A Safe Rescue

Here are some tips to ensure an "unsung hero's" safe return. First of all, remember that you shouldn't go in a burning room or building solo if you can help it. Have someone wait for you outside. Otherwise, you could become a "hurt hero." And always call for professional help first! If possible, wait until the fire truck arrives. Firefighters know how to get in and out of a burning building much better than you do. They also have the equipment to handle electrical fires, wood-burning fires, and chemical fires—and they know how to use it!

> **First Things First**
> If you're caught in a fire, the first thing you should do is cover your face with a wet towel, a piece of cloth, your shirt, or anything else you can find to help reduce the inhalation of smoke. You cannot save a life or yourself if you are overcome with smoke.

But, if you can't possibly wait for help, there are some safety measures you can take. If the smoke in a room is not coming from a full-blown fire, take several deep breaths before entering. Then, holding your breath, enter and pull the victim outside. If smoke is heavy, determine whether it's circling the ceiling (which is usually the case because heat and warm air rise) or hanging around the floor (which can occur in chemical fires). Then enter the room accordingly. Crouch if the smoke is high. Keep your head straight up and tall if it's low.

By the time you and the victim are out in the fresh air, the fire department should have arrived—hopefully! Don't further compromise yourself by trying to put out the fire on your own. Remember, the victim suffered from smoke inhalation, and it is possible you could be injured too. Let the professionals do their jobs.

If help is not yet on the scene, forget the building and concentrate on the survivors. If someone's clothing is on fire, he or she should use the "stop, drop, and roll" method:

1. Stop in your tracks.

2. Drop to the ground.

3. Roll on the ground in attempt to smother the flames.

The Least You Need to Know

➤ Smoke inhalation occurs from minor fires, such as stovetop fires and improperly vented fireplaces.

➤ Minor symptoms include coughing and red eyes.

➤ Major symptoms include difficulty breathing, choking, and (ultimately) unconsciousness.

➤ Call for help before you do anything else.

➤ Make sure you take several deep breaths before entering the smoke-filled area yourself. Hold your breath as you pull the victim out.

➤ If the victim is unconscious, check for vital signs and then the ABCs of first aid care: Make sure that Airways are clear, Breathing is regular, and Circulation is normal. (See Chapter 1 for more information.)

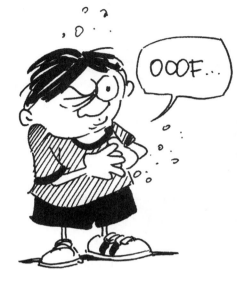

Chapter 27

Stomach Aches, Diarrhea, Indigestion, and Other Digestive Problems

In This Chapter

➤ Relief from constipation

➤ Stopping diarrhea in its tracks

➤ Is it gas... or something more serious?

➤ What heartburn is—and how to prevent it

➤ Discovering ulcer cures

➤ Coping with an appendicitis emergency

Stomach problems occur in as many shapes and sizes as the stomachs they affect. Whether the sufferer's problem is a minor attack of gas or the "runs," or something more serious like an ulcer or a hernia, there is first aid care that can help.

Although not every condition in this chapter is an emergency, all of them can cause, at the very least, discomfort. And, because some conditions can be symptomatic of something serious, something that can make the difference between life and death, it's important to recognize all of the symptoms ...and know what to do.

The *digestive system* is more than your stomach, a "rolled up" tube of intestines, and your rectum. To help you understand why stomachs can have acid upsets, stools can be watery, and hemorrhoids can hurt, here's the "soups to nuts" on how the system works:

1. You put some food in your mouth.

2. Your *saliva glands* produce fluid that "softens" the food so that you can chew the food into small pieces more easily.

3. The "lumps" of food go down your throat (or *esophagus*).

4. The semi-digested food moves through your *stomach*. Water and other fluids pass right through the stomach's wall to hungry blood cells.

5. The semi-digested food is broken down even more by *gastric juices* in the stomach.

6. The food passes through the coiled up *small intestine*, which is divided into three parts: the *duodenum, jejunum,* and the *ileum*.

7. As food passes through each part of the small intestine, it gets more and more broken up and digested—helped along by the *digestive enzymes* produced in the *pancreas*.

8. The food is made even more digestible by *bile* produced in the *liver* and stored in the *gall bladder*. The gall bladder releases its store of bile as the food enters the duodenum.

9. After the broken down food has journeyed through the small intestine, it is digested. All that remains is a few fragments of food and fluid, left-over bile, bacteria, and waste—which then enters the *large intestine*.

10. The large intestine (or *colon*) moves the waste along for elimination. The good bacteria in the large intestine break down any remaining food (except for high fiber foods which pass out of the body undigested). The fluid that journeys with it passes through the colon walls, leaving a semi-soft mass called *stool*.

11. The stool is pushed out through the *rectum,* the *anal canal,* and the *anus*.

From a chocolate chip cookie to a tangerine, the process is the same. By the time the food you've eaten is eliminated, the taste of that cookie or fruit is a memory …which you might want to immediately make reality once again!

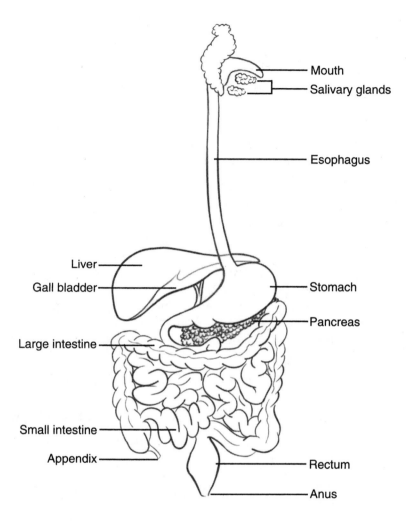

The digestive system.

- Mouth
- Salivary glands
- Esophagus
- Liver
- Gall bladder
- Stomach
- Pancreas
- Large intestine
- Small intestine
- Appendix
- Rectum
- Anus

Treating Diarrhea

Diarrhea. The condition that makes a common denominator of us all. Everyone, at some time in his or her life, has had a bout of the "runs"—hopefully in situations where a bathroom was nearby.

Minor cases of the runs can be the result of:

➤ Overeating

➤ Nerves

➤ Minor viral infections

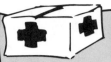

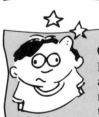

➤ Alcohol overindulgence

➤ A side effect of medication

➤ Eating food that's just begun to spoil

➤ Lactose intolerance (which means your stomach's digestive acids lack the enzyme that will properly digest the sugar in milk, causing gas, heartburn, and diarrhea)

➤ Taking too many antacids (which translates into too much magnesium and, ultimately, watery stools)

Unless the sufferer is lactose intolerant (in which case you should change to a lactose-free milk) or takes too many antacids (in which case he or she should cut down), there's little you need to do but let "nature take its course." However, to ensure someone with diarrhea is as comfortable as possible and that there are no side effects, follow these steps:

1. Stop all food until the bout of diarrhea is past. (One full day is recommended.) This gives an irritated digestive system a chance to calm down.

2. Offer the person having the problem liquids instead of solids. The liquids help hydrate the body, replacing liquids lost during the bout of diarrhea. Stick with clear liquids, such as apple juice and 7-Up, and avoid acidic orange juice and caffeinated cola products. (These other liquids are also good: chicken and beef broth, gelatin dissolved in warm water, and herbal teas.)

3. You can also give the sufferer an anti-diarrheal medication, such as Pepto-Bismol, Kaopectate, or Immodium.

4. If the bout of diarrhea stops during the first 24 hours, you can start giving the ill person solid foods. But go easy. The digestive tract is still sensitive! You might try hot cereal, toast, soft-boiled eggs, or chicken soup.

5. There are times when it's wise to call a doctor, even if the problem is only mild diarrhea. If the diarrhea is accompanied by a high fever and severe cramps that don't subside, it could be a sign of something serious. Call your physician for guidance!

Minor diarrhea is easily cured and a call to the doctor or the emergency room is usually not necessary. But there are times when diarrhea can signal more serious illnesses—or lead to illness itself. These sections describe situations you should be mindful of, so you know when to seek expert care.

"Montezuma's Revenge"

The legend has it that when the Spaniards attacked and horribly massacred the Aztecs in Mexico, they were left a vengeful legacy: an illness that involved terrible diarrhea, nausea, stomach cramps, and vomiting. Named after Montezuma, the King of the Aztecs, this "revenge" for the massacre can easily befall any tourist visiting Mexico today. The symptoms of "Montezuma's Revenge" are similar to those of food poisoning (see Chapter 22). However, rather than food, it involves parasites or bacteria in the water. While the enzymes in the digestive systems of Mexicans (and people of other Caribbean cultures) have long ago adapted to this water, tourists from Canada and the United States are not so lucky. If "tainted" water is swallowed, either from brushing one's teeth, showering, eating food washed in regular water, or drinks made with tainted ice cubes, tourists can easily succumb to a terrible attack of diarrhea. If you are a tourist from the states, you should also avoid unpeeled fruits, salads, and raw vegetables. These too can be "tainted."

> **First Things First**
> Today there are prescription antibiotics that travelers can take before they partake to prevent Montezuma's Revenge. The good news is that it gives you the freedom to eat and drink what you want. The bad news is that it can cause such side effects as drowsiness, headaches, nausea, and rashes.

If it's not treated, "Montezuma's Revenge" can cause dehydration, severe weakness, and possible shock. The best protection against getting it in the first place is to use bottled water in any country where tainted water might be a problem.

Dehydration

Diarrhea can cause dehydration. Your body can also become dehydrated from too much vomiting and a lack of drinking water, especially on a hot summer day.

The food you eat and the liquid you drink on a daily basis comes to about three or four liters or one gallon of fluid. When this fluid reaches the intestines, approximately eight ounces is eliminated as a bowel movement. The rest is either eliminated in your urine or absorbed into your body.

When you have diarrhea, the solids become watery. And if you're going to the bathroom five or six times a day, you're losing a lot more liquid than you should. It's easy to see how your body could become dehydrated.

Most bouts of minor dehydration can be handled by slowly drinking liquids. But, unfortunately, dehydration can become serious quickly. Dehydration attacks the filtering system of the kidneys, "drying out" the water in our bodies that help our vital fluids run smoothly so that our cells can be replenished and our toxins eliminated. When diarrhea continues for more than 24 hours, the loss of water and fluids can reach dangerous levels.

Before You Put the Band-Aid On

It's good to sip any liquid if you have a minor case of dehydration. "Sports drinks," such as Snapple's K-10 and Gatorade, work even better because they contain glucose and potassium, which are vital nutrients your body needs for good health—and which are lost when you become dehydrated. However, adults who are dehydrated will find quicker results if they alternate a "sports drink" with water and juice. Children will do better with Pedialyte, a "dehydration" brew made specifically for youngsters. And the World Health Organization (WHO) makes rehydration powders that are more balanced, but are not as tasty, as Gatorade.

Signs of dehydration include:

Extreme drowsiness	Weakness
Clammy skin and chills	Dizziness
Rough, lackluster skin that "tents" or "sags" when pulled	Being able to eliminate only small quantities of dark urine
An inability to urinate	Eventual unconsciousness

If someone is dehydrated, have him or her sip water, not gulp it down. The stomach cannot handle too much water—and the person who's ill will end up vomiting the water, causing even more dehydration. Dehydration becomes more and more serious very quickly. Hospital treatment is imperative if you suspect dehydration. The treatment for serious dehydration is intravenous fluid intake—which only a hospital can supply.

Irritable Bowel Syndrome

The bad news about Irritable Bowel Syndrome (IBS) is that there's no one thing you can point to and say, "Ah ha, there's the culprit: Irritable Bowel Syndrome." We still aren't sure why some people come down with IBS and others don't.

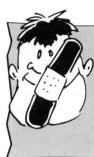

Before You Put the Band-Aid On

Although studies are still relatively recent, scientists and nutritionists are beginning to find a possible "root" for IBS: a leaky gut. In other words, the intestines are not functioning properly and the enzymes are not doing their job. This can be the result of a deficiency in "good" bacteria, poor diet, and stress.

The good news, however, is that if IBS is diagnosed, it means that much more serious conditions, such as colitis, ulcers, gallbladder disease, and other diseases have been ruled out. IBS is essentially a digestive system that's gone awry. The intestines have trouble moving food along and out of the body. This translates into abdominal cramps and pain, followed by diarrhea (or, in some cases, constipation) that is relieved after you go to the bathroom—only to return a few hours later.

IBS is not an emergency situation. However, there are some first aid treatments that can make the condition more bearable and, perhaps, alleviate the symptoms:

➤ Cut out high-fat foods. Studies have found fat linked to IBS.

➤ Add more fiber to your diet. The fiber can help tame an "angry" digestive tract.

➤ Avoid spicy foods. They can irritate the bowel even more.

➤ Try an antispasmodic medication, under a doctor's supervision. When stomach pain is bad, this medication can relax the intestine's muscles. Only one brand that stops cramping is sold over-the-counter: Donnagel. All the others are sold by prescription only.

Colitis

Similar to IBS, colitis is officially "an inflammation of the colon." With colitis, the digestive system can be working properly—until it reaches the large intestine (or colon). Food and liquid are properly digested and used by the body. The pancreas has sent in the proper enzymes to further break up food and liquid particles and send the food on its way to all the parts of the body. The liver has sent in bile to dissolve fat and make the food "palatable" for absorption. By the time fluids and food have reached the large intestine, all that remains is some left-over bile and rejected bacteria—ready to be eliminated as stool.

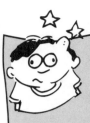

Ouch!
If a sufferer's diarrhea is combined with severe abdominal pain or bloody, dark stool and fever, get help as soon as you can. Stomach pain can signal appendicitis, a hernia, or even a possible heart attack (covered in Chapter 17). A bloody, dark stool can mean internal bleeding. Fever can signal a viral infection, bacterial infection, or a perforation (rupture) of the intestinal wall and can lead to convulsions or shock. (See Chapter 13 for more information.)

But, if the colon becomes inflamed, irritated, or sore, the stool that is created might not be "true to form." The stool is watery and a bad case of watery diarrhea, (sometimes containing blood from the irritated colon's lining) is the result. The diarrhea can be followed or preceded by bouts of constipation.

Colitis can be triggered by stress. Although not an emergency, it can lead to dehydration and an imbalanced, weakened digestive system.

If someone has colitis, he or she should absolutely be under a physician's care and be aware of the following:

➤ Diet should be higher in fiber; eating an apple every day is a good idea.

➤ Relaxation techniques should be encouraged.

➤ The doctor can prescribe medication that can help reduce the symptoms.

Relief from Constipation

Just as everyone has had at least one bout of diarrhea in their lives, so, too, has everyone been constipated on occasion.

In technical terms, constipation is the opposite of diarrhea. It means that your colon is not getting the signal to contract and push out waste.

What causes constipation? A number of things, including:

Lack of exercise

Drinking too little water

Side-effects of medications

Ignoring the need to go to the bathroom

Lack of fiber in your diet

Too much iron

A frantic lifestyle

The first sign of constipation is obvious: not going to the bathroom on a regular basis. (This varies among individuals. For some people, regular is daily; for others, it's every other day. And for still other, it might be every third day.) There are other signs as well:

A week goes by before one finds relief

The need to strain to move the bowels

Hemorrhoids develop

Stools are small and hard

Bright, red blood on the surface of the stools

A full, bloated, and gassy feeling

Regular Treatment

Normally, constipation can be taken care of at home, without emergency care. Here are some tips for relief:

➤ Eat more raw fruits and vegetables. High fiber helps your colon contract, helping you go to the bathroom.

➤ Use a fiber product such as Metamucil biscuits or Citrucel every morning to increase fiber intake.

➤ Exercise! A good walk or time on the NordicTrak stimulates the colon.

➤ Drink eight to twelve glasses of water, herb tea, or non-caffeinated drinks every day. Fluids keep the digestive system humming.

➤ Don't take an iron pill unless instructed by your physician. A multivitamin/mineral supplement ensures that you get the nutrients you need without the excess iron that can cause constipation.

➤ Ask your physician about any medication you are taking. Certain antidepressants, high blood pressure pills, and pain relievers can cause constipation by blocking the chemical that signals the brain to tell the colon to "push!"

➤ Don't take over-the-counter laxatives on a regular basis. They can become habit-forming, preventing you from having a bowel movement *without* them. They can also damage the colon in the long run.

Ouch!
If you decide to use a powdered fiber product like Metamucil, make sure you dissolve the instructed amount in enough water. If you don't take enough fluid with the "bulk," you can wind up even more constipated!

First Aids
Diverticulitis is a condition in which tiny pieces of food get "trapped" in the folds of the intestines, causing irritation, digestive problems, and bleeding from the large intestine.

Crohn's disease is an inflammation of the ileum section of the small intestine (and can often include the large intestine colon as well). It is usually combined with small bumps, polyps, or lumps on the intestinal wall and changes in bowel movement, from constipation to bloody diarrhea.

If someone's constipation continues for more than two weeks (even after you've tried normal, everyday remedies), it's time to see the doctor.

Constipation that doesn't heal itself can signal some serious conditions, such as colon cancer, colitis, Irritable Bowel Syndrome (IBS), diverticulitis, or Crohn's disease. If constipation is combined with blood and stomach pain, see a doctor to check for these things.

Hemorrhoid Pain, Burn, and Itching

Hemorrhoids are about as common as bouts of minor constipation. From print ads to television ads, we've all learned how to treat the pain, burning, and itching that's associated with this common ailment.

Sure, we all know the general vicinity of these ubiquitous, difficult-to-spell "things," but do you really know exactly what hemorrhoids are?

Right inside the anus are blood vessels that act almost as inflated "air bags." They form a secure covering around the anus, preventing gas, stool, and air from leaking into the rectum. However, these "air bag" blood vessels can easily become inflamed, swollen, and droopy from too much straining during a bowel movement. These droopy, swollen, inflamed blood vessels are *hemorrhoids*.

Signs of Hemorrhoids

Hemorrhoids are hardly a first aid emergency, but they can cause discomfort and inconvenience at the worst times. Here are some of the symptoms that signal hemorrhoids and the need for relief:

➤ Itchiness in the rectum and anal area

➤ Burning pain, especially after a bowel movement

➤ Bright red blood on the surface of stool or on the toilet paper

➤ Swollen anus

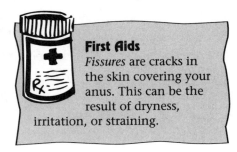

First Aids
Fissures are cracks in the skin covering your anus. This can be the result of dryness, irritation, or straining.

Ninety percent of the people doctors see with these symptoms have hemorrhoids. These symptoms also can mean fissures, ulcerative colitis, a fungus, a serious condition in another area of your digestive system, a cyst or lump, or a sexually transmitted disease. If you have any of the above symptoms, you should see your doctor to rule out anything dangerous.

Hemorrhoid Relief

Everyone knows that hemorrhoids cause an itching, burning feeling. Even if you have never experienced it yourself, you still know all about it thanks to television ads and the print media.

Although almost a cliché, hemorrhoids are no laughing matter. They can cause a great deal of discomfort, and in severe cases, they might have to be surgically removed. But surgery is a last-ditch effort. There's much you can do before to find relief. Here are some first aid suggestions:

> ➤ Over-the-counter ointments can reduce the swelling and burning of hemorrhoids; they also provide lubrication, which makes it easier to have a bowel movement.

> ➤ Eating more fiber and drinking powdered fiber products, such as Metamucil, will also help relieve the straining that comes from constipation.

> ➤ An over-the-counter stool softener can ease the pain.

> ➤ Drink lots of water, at least eight glasses a day. Water also keeps stool from getting too hard and, consequently, difficult to eliminate.

> ➤ Reduce the amount of coffee you drink. Coffee beans contain oil that, ground and made into a powder, can irritate the anus as the liquid coffee waste is eliminated from the body.

> ➤ Use good hygiene. Wash the area with a washcloth and water in the shower or bath.

First Aids
Note that a *stool softener* is not a *laxative*. The softener is exactly what it sounds like; it makes the actual stool softer. Laxatives, on the other hand, will make you feel the urge to go to the bathroom. They are fine to take for constipation on a very occasional basis, but people can become dependent on them, unable to go to the bathroom without one. Furthermore, too many laxatives can be hazardous to your health because they can cause dehydration.

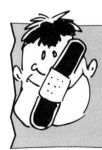

Before You Put the Band-Aid On

Believe it or not, plain old inexpensive petroleum jelly can do the job when it comes to hemorrhoids. Applying a small amount whenever you feel that burning or itching feeling can help relieve the pain.

Indigestion, Heartburn, and Ulcers

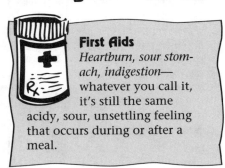

First Aids
Heartburn, sour stomach, indigestion— whatever you call it, it's still the same acidy, sour, unsettling feeling that occurs during or after a meal.

There you are, sitting with your family and enjoying a celebration dinner at the best restaurant in town. As you blow out the candle and dip into the ice cream surprise, you suddenly feel a pang. Ouch! The bitter, queasy taste of heartburn hits. You say your excuses and go off to the bathroom, silently berating yourself for eating that shallot, hot pepper, and garlic sauce.

It might not happen exactly that way, but when heartburn hits, it knows no bounds, no excuses, and no options.

The Ins and Outs of Heartburn

More than 40 million Americans suffer from heartburn on occasion, that sour feeling that occurs when stomach acid splashes back up into the esophagus.

At the point where the esophagus and the stomach meet is a muscle called the lower esophageal sphincter (LES). This muscle acts like a trap door, opening to let food into the stomach, then closing up tight to prevent the food from coming out.

There are certain actions that can irritate and reopen the LES, spilling stomach acid back into the esophagus and creating heartburn. These include:

➤ Eating spicy, fatty, sour, or minty foods that don't agree with you

➤ Overindulging during a meal

➤ Being overweight

➤ Drinking too much coffee or alcohol

➤ Smoking cigarettes

➤ Taking some medications, including unbuffered aspirin

➤ Wearing belts and waistbands that are too tight

➤ Being pregnant

➤ Taking birth control pills

Treating Heartburn

Taking over-the-counter antacids is the most common treatment for heartburn—and, unless you are taking a medication that contradicts the alkaline in antacids—they usually work fast.

However, today there are also preventative medications on the market that not only neutralize the acid that creeps back up, but reduce the amount of acid that is made. These include the two best-selling prescription medications, Tagamet and Zantac (which are now sold over-the-counter). These medications block acid in your stomach and are successful for people with ulcers.

Both Tagamet and Zantac are called H2 Antagonists. You can get milder forms of these medications as well. These milder over-the-counter pills need to be taken an hour before a spicy meal to be effective.

However, these medications need time to work and if you are having an attack of indigestion or heartburn *now*, the best bet is still an antacid.

Ouch!
Although heartburn is a common ailment, it can also signal something more serious: a heart attack. Many people who come into an emergency room with what they think is simply a bad case of indigestion could be having more serious problems. If you feel an intense, unrelenting bout of heartburn, go to a doctor—fast!

You can also try to prevent heartburn with non-medication treatment tricks. Here are some suggestions:

➤ Eat several small meals during the day instead of three big ones.

➤ Avoid spicy food, alcohol, coffee, and any other foods that can irritate your digestive tract.

➤ Eat your last meal several hours before you go to sleep. (This gives your body a chance to completely digest the food.)

➤ Eat slowly and put the fork down between bites. (This too helps you digest foods more easily.)

➤ Sleep with your head and upper torso raised about six inches. A foam wedge works well.

➤ Learn to relax. The less stress you feel, the better your entire body will work.

If antacids aren't available and someone is experiencing a bout of heartburn, give him or her one half of a cup or less of skim milk (only if the person does not have any problems with meat or dairy; for some people, eating protein creates a condition that is somewhere between an ulcer and heartburn). If there are no problems with ingesting protein, the skim milk can be an effective antacid substitute for heartburn or ulcers because it helps neutralize the acid. Further, skim milk contains no fat, which can be an irritant.

First Things First
Another easy heartburn antidote is deep breathing. The more you relax your body, the less likely it is that the "trap door" will let acid leak back out.

The key is to drink a small enough amount to work, but not enough to "splash up." If skim milk isn't available, even a glass of water might help.

Whether you sip skim milk or water, it's important to remember one key thing: sit up for at least 30 minutes after you've sipped the liquid. This position will help the liquid do its "magic."

Ulcer Understanding

The main difference between an ulcer and indigestion is that the former is often more serious than the latter. However, indigestion can be a warning sign of an ulcer (although not in every person). In other words, heartburn/sour stomach/indigestion can be a symptom of an ulcer, a condition in which the normal stomach lining breaks down, revealing unprotected tissue that is irritated by stomach acid. Or it can signal plain old indigestion.

An ulcer looks like a cluster of painful sores on the inner lining of the stomach. An ulcer can bleed and cause a great deal of pain, including cramps, indigestion, and severe heartburn.

Cause and Effect: An Up-To-The-Minute Ulcer Newsflash

For years, diet was blamed as much for ulcers as it was for heartburn. No more. A change in diet will not cure your ulcer, but it can still help. Scientists have isolated a bacteria called *Helicobacterpylori (H. pylori)* as the cause of some of these painful sores. Many—but not all—ulcers are now considered an infection like influenza, strep throat, and the common cold.

What's interesting is the fact that about 50 percent of us carry the *H. pylori* bacteria in our stomachs and intestines but have no reaction. Unfortunately, the other 50 percent's immune systems cannot keep *H. pylori* quiet. They have ulcers.

If your heartburn is long-term and severe, and you experience pain in your stomach or intestines, make an appointment with your doctor. Ulcers don't usually constitute life-and-death emergencies unless they bleed—but they can make a daily routine pretty miserable!

The best treatment for ulcers is the same acid blockers used for heartburn, either in over-the-counter formulas or in the stronger prescription ones, such as Tagamet and Zantac.

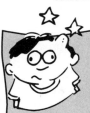

Ouch!
As with any medication, acid blockers also can have side-effects in some people. Headaches, drowsiness, diarrhea, gas, and dizziness are the most common. However, these symptoms usually disappear within a few days. You also should check with your doctor about combining acid blockers with other medications; certain combos can cause adverse reactions.

Researchers have also discovered that certain antibiotics or a regimen of acid blockers combined with plain old Pepto-Bismol can get rid of *H. pylori* in a matter of weeks in most cases.

"Flu-ing" the Coop

Stomach flus are as much a part of our lives as, well, tooth decay and sore throats.

Stomach flu can be a "24-hour" bug or an infection that lasts for a few days. Signs of stomach flu include:

Bouts of diarrhea	Chills and clammy skin
Weakness	Aches and pains
Stomach cramps	Nausea and vomiting

Stomach flus are caused by a virus which, instead of heading, say, for the throat or lungs, lodges in your digestive tract.

Our immune systems, made up of ever vigilant antibodies and other "warrior" cells, are designed to "catch" these alien invaders called viruses, before they sneak through the cell wall. But sometimes a new strain gets past the warriors and, before you can say "I'm nauseous!," the virus cells grow.

Luckily, our immune systems usually discover what's up and, before you can say "I'm feeling better!," they've stopped the virus from growing out of hand. This is especially true for common strains of flu. Eventually, even with a slight mutation, our immune system recognizes the virus for what it is: stomach flu—as it leads our body to victory.

> **First Aids**
> A *virus* is really an unfinished cell. Because it needs a full-fledged, functioning cell to exist, it "invades" a healthy cell and begins to do its dirty work, changing the healthy cell into a sick "virus" cell. This virus cell, in turn, is now cleverly disguised as a healthy cell. It can easily invade another cell, and another cell, and so on.

Stomach flus are more inconvenient than dangerous. Follow the same first aid treatment you would for diarrhea (earlier in this chapter) or nausea (see Chapter 22). If a stomach flu continues for more than two or three days and it is combined with high fever, make an appointment to see your physician. You may need a prescription medication to get rid of the viral infection.

Help! Appendicitis!

Beware of stomach pain that remains in the lower right side of your stomach, especially if this area feels tender when gently pressed.

Appendicitis can strike at any time. At first, it looks like simple diarrhea or a minor stomach flu, but the symptoms get worse and the pain intensifies. The nausea doesn't go away. If someone has the following symptoms get him or her to an emergency room quickly:

Fever

Nausea and inability to eat

Intense pain in the lower right side of the stomach

Constipation

Although a blood test will ultimately provide the proof, it's better to be safe than sorry. An infected, inflamed appendix will just get larger and larger until it bursts. It *must* be removed under anesthesia as soon as possible.

A ruptured (or burst) appendix can spread infection throughout your body. And, yes, people can still die from the blood poisoning caused by a ruptured appendix.

Unfortunately, unless you are a trained surgeon, there's not much you can do for an appendicitis attack. The most important thing is to get help as fast as possible. And, while you're waiting keep the patient as comfortable as possible:

➤ Cover him or her with a loose blanket

➤ Provide water if he or she wants it

➤ Warm tea can also help soothe the pain

➤ Watch for symptoms of shock. If necessary, treat for this condition while you wait for help to arrive. (See Chapter 3 for first aid treatment for shock.)

➤ Do *not* give the person food. It can cause even more pain and create complications!

➤ Do *not* offer any medication. Antacids will have no effect and aspirin might increase the nausea.

Before You Put the Band-Aid On

Because appendicitis can attack so suddenly without any warning, astronauts have their appendixes removed before a space launch…just in case.

We might live quite happily today without our appendixes, but, long ago, in primitive times, they had a real reason to be. Once upon a time, this worm-like organ was a storage pouch that kept bacteria ready to help digest the inedible leafs and greens that made up our ancestors' diets.

The Least You Need to Know

➤ Stomach upsets are rarely traumatic, unless they are a symptom of a heart attack or an appendicitis attack.

➤ If someone is suffering from diarrhea, avoid solid foods for a day.

➤ Avoid the dehydration that can come with diarrhea by drinking plenty of fluids.

➤ Heartburn can often be prevented by living a healthier lifestyle.

➤ Ulcers can be caused by a specific bacteria, and medication is necessary to destroy it.

➤ Hemorrhoids are extremely common. They are caused by straining during a bowel movement. A diet rich in fiber and a stool softener can help.

➤ For constipation, try eating fiber and powdered fiber products daily.

➤ If you have painful or persistent indigestion, go to a hospital. Chances are, you just ate too much, but it can be a sign of a heart attack.

➤ Appendicitis symptoms include tenderness and pain on the lower-right side of the stomach. The only treatment for appendicitis is surgery; go to the emergency room immediately.

Part 3
First Aid for Women

Ever since the first woman burned the first bra, the women's movement has called for equality between the sexes. And, of course, equality is an undeniable truth. When it comes to work, personal issues, athletics, stamina, and family life, women are the equal to men in every way (and, as some would argue, superior!).

But you can be equal (read: superior) and different at the same time. And, as the birds and the bees would be the first to say, "Viva la différence!"

These differences are physical, which means they sometimes necessitate different first aid know-how. The problems range from menstrual cramps to pregnancy complications, from cystitis to yeast infections. The important thing is to know what to do to avoid the problem—or, for those conditions that are unavoidable, how to lessen the discomfort. Because of these physical differences, we've devoted an entire part to "women only" and their particular first aid needs.

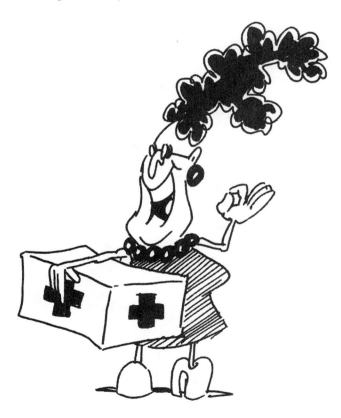

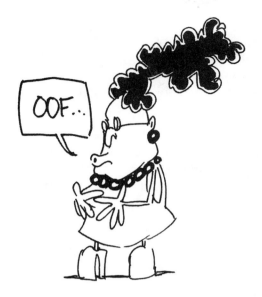

Common Come-and-Go Conditions

Although men can also get cystitis, urinary tract infections, and discomfort in their genitals, women are the primary targets for these common ailments. Why? Because a woman's hormonal balance changes each month. Her reproductive system's job makes her more vulnerable to germs and complications.

This chapter discusses some of the common "come-and-go" conditions that almost every woman experiences at some time in her life.

Tender Breasts

Many women know that their period (menstruation) is due because of one factor: their breasts start to hurt. This pain varies from woman to woman, depending on each one's hormonal balance. For some women, this pain is worse than for others, and for some women, the pain begins two weeks before the actual menstrual flow and doesn't ebb until the period begins.

Breast tenderness is believed to be caused by a natural excess of female hormones that generally occurs at a certain time during the monthly cycle. These hormones include estrogen, progesterone, and prolactin. This monthly fluctuation creates some havoc in the body, including fluid retention, bloating, and swelling. Fluid retention in the breasts can make them tender.

There are other reasons for breast tenderness that have less to do with hormones and menstrual cycles—and everything to do with daily habits. These reasons can include:

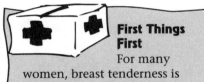

First Things First

For many women, breast tenderness is worse during perimenopause, the five to ten years before menopause actually takes place. During this time, hormones are subtly beginning to change. Fluctuations in menstrual flow, PMS symptoms, and mood swings begin.

➤ Inactivity among the couch potato set

➤ Prolonged emotional distress

➤ Stress at home, on the job, or within relationships

➤ Too much salt in the diet

➤ Obesity

➤ Too much coffee, soda, or other caffeinated drinks

➤ A high-fat diet

Whatever a woman's age, these factors can escalate breast tenderness. The best advice is prevention. Some of the best things you can do to ease your pain are to:

➤ Exercise before you start getting premenstrual symptoms. Walking, swimming, or doing low-impact aerobics (wearing a good sports bra) three times a week will help ease monthly discomfort.

➤ Think soft. Put a small pad of soft lamb's wool in your bra cup. You can purchase small amounts in a medical supply store or even in a pet shop!

➤ Take two ibuprofen tablets (such as Motrin or Advil) to lessen swelling of the breasts.

➤ Adjust your hormone replacement therapy if you are presently under a physician's care for menopause. Your doctor can adjust the progesterone for the few days you are experiencing breast tenderness.

➤ Apply ice packs or cold compresses for approximately fifteen minutes at a time.

➤ Change your diet. Stay away from high-fat, refined sugar, and salt.

The Uncomfortable Burn of Cystitis

Nicknamed the "Honeymoon Disease," urinary tract infection (UTI) or *cystitis* has long been associated with too much …well, you get the picture. However, in reality, cystitis is an infection that is caused by any number of things and is considered by physicians to be as common as the cold. And, as it does with the common cold, your immune system has a lot to do with whether or not you get urinary tract infections—as well as with reoccurrence.

The lower urinary tract consists of the genitals, the urethra leading to the bladder, and the bladder itself. This is an ideal site for bacteria to grow. It is moist, mucousy, and warm—an environment that bacteria finds impossible to resist.

Furthermore, each woman's immune systems makes her vulnerable to different things. Why do some people get certain diseases and others get off scot-free? Each immune system, in addition to a genetic predisposition, has a lot to do with it. Germs not easily "warded off" by the immune system's "warrior" antibodies can cause flu, colds, or urinary tract infections. And, because stress can weaken the immune system, too much angst and anxiety can also create the perfect environment for UTI.

> **First Aids**
> *Escherichia coli,* or E-coli as it is called for short, is the bacteria that causes 90 percent of all urinary tract infections. It is the same bacteria found in the colon and the rectum—which are only a short "hop" from the woman's urinary tract.

The symptoms of cystitis, or UTI, are not subtle. They can include:

➤ A burning sensation when you urinate

➤ An urgency to urinate—maybe within half an hour of when you last did so

➤ Difficulty urinating

➤ Soreness and a feeling of "fullness" in your bladder or stomach area

➤ Blood in the urine

You can alleviate some of the more uncomfortable symptoms by trying the following:

➤ Sit in a shallow "sitz" bath of warm water with a sprinkle of baking soda to soothe the burning feeling.

➤ Drink eight to ten glasses of water a day to "flush" away bacteria in your bladder.

➤ Avoid sex until the infection has passed. Both sexual activity and most contraceptives (including IUDs, sponges, diaphragms, foam, and certain condoms) can irritate already inflamed tissue.

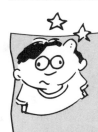

Ouch!
If your physician prescribes Pyridium to help alleviate your pain, bloating, and urgent need to urinate, take note. Pyridium turns your urine red—but it is harmless!

➤ Eat bland foods. Acidic foods such as citrus fruits, pineapple, strawberries, liquor, coffee, chocolate, apples, tea, tomatoes, and vinegar will make the irritation worse.

➤ Take acetaminophen (Tylenol) if the condition is very painful. Over-the-counter Cysotex and prescription-only Pyridium also help relieve the pain, the bloating, and the desperate need to urinate.

Before You Put the Band-Aid On

Although 20 percent of all women get urinary tract infections, only five percent of all men get them. A man's anatomy makes it more difficult for E-coli germs to travel from the rectum to the urethra and the bladder. A man's prostate gland also secretes a strong bacteria-fighting substance. UTIs are so rare in men that, if a man shows any symptoms, he should go to the doctor immediately. It can signal a serious condition, such as prostate cancer or diabetes.

Treating UTI

The method of treatment for cystitis is antibiotics. If the results of a urinalysis come back positive, your physician will most likely prescribe Bactrim or Septra for three days. Seven used to be the magic number when it came to UTI antibiotic routines. The prescribed medications had to be taken for seven days—or the infection would come back. No more. Today, physicians know that a three-day regime is just as effective—with less chance of the common side-effects of antibiotics: upset stomach, nausea, yeast infection, and the "gobbling up" of "good bacteria" along with the bad.

Many urinary tract infections reoccur. Most of these reoccurring infections are the result of a "germ friendly" bladder or a bacteria resistant to the particular antibiotic you were taking. However, sometimes reoccurring UTI can signal a serious condition such as kidney stones, urinary tract obstructions, bladder dysfunction, diabetes, or cancer. If you have cystitis more than twice within six months, or three to four infections within a year, you should be tested for these other ailments.

Prevention Is More Than Half the Cure

You can help prevent reoccurring infections with a few easy-to-follow hints:

➤ *Face forward.* Always wipe from front to back when you go to the bathroom. It will help keep E-coli bacteria away from your urinary tract.

➤ *Cleanliness is next to godliness.* As with all first aid treatments, washing your hands before performing any task will help keep germs at bay. Personal hygiene is crucial—especially before and after you've inserted a tampon, before and after you've had sex, and after you've gone to the bathroom.

➤ *Safe sex.* One prime element of sexual relationships in today's world, contraceptives can promote UTI. Make sure your diaphragm is positioned properly and does not obstruct the bladder. Avoid any spermicides that have caused cystitis previously. And note that some jellies kill "good bacteria" along with sperm. A condom, for many reasons, is the best contraceptive for safe sex.

➤ *Wet blanket.* Urinary tract infections thrive in dampness. Change that wet bathing suit as soon as you can. Avoid tight pants and panty hose that do not "breathe." Cotton undies are best.

➤ *Crave the wave.* Studies have found that cranberry juice really works in inhibiting UTI. It creates a "slippery environment" in your urinary tract, which keeps E-coli and other "bad" germs from adhering to its walls. For those of you on a diet, health stores have cranberry juice tablets with the same power minus the calories.

➤ *The silent passage.* Menopause decreases the amount of estrogen your body produces. This, in turn, creates a drier vagina and urethra—which are much more vulnerable to becoming irritated, inflamed, and susceptible to UTI. But estrogen cream and estrogen replacement therapy helps prevent UTI by lubricating the dry areas.

➤ *Drink plenty of water.* Six to eight glasses every day can help "flush" your system.

➤ *Take lots of breaks.* Get up from your desk several times a day. Sitting all day without relieving yourself gives bacteria time to set up shop.

Ouch!
Although new studies have shown that cranberry juice may prevent cystitis, other studies have shown that when an infection is in place, the acidity of the juice may escalate the condition, providing a hostile environment perfect for "bad germs" to live. The moral? Take cranberry juice for prevention only.

Menstrual Problems

Now even the most conservative physicians no longer believe that PMS is "all in the head." Problems that crop up two weeks before you start menstruating and those that occur during your period are very real. Here are the more common problems—and what you can do about them.

Coping with PMS

Surveys have found that as many as 60 percent of all women suffer from symptoms of premenstrual syndrome (or PMS) 10–15 days before the onset of menstruation. In some women, PMS continues for two to three days during menstruation.

The cause of PMS is due to changes in hormone secretion during the latter two weeks of a woman's cycle. It can be made worse by stress, improper rest, or too little or too much exercise (all of which affect hormones greatly). A salty, spicy diet (which makes for water retention and, in turn, uncomfortable bloating, swelling, and pressure on nerves, joints, and organs) also affects PMS.

Symptoms of PMS include:

Anxiety and irritability	Headaches
Mood swings	Fatigue
Weight gain	Breast tenderness
Sugar cravings	Lower back pain
Cramps	Nausea
Depression	Oily skin and skin eruptions
Stomach bloating	

Chances are you won't suffer from all these symptoms, but you'll feel enough of them if you have PMS to make those days before your period uncomfortable.

You can avoid severe PMS symptoms by following these some common-sense guidelines:

➤ Eat a sensible diet that emphasizes fresh vegetables and fruit, fish, whole grain cereals, and bread. Avoid salty, spicy foods, especially in the third and fourth week of your cycle.

➤ Get a good night's sleep. If necessary, drink some "Sleepy Time" herbal tea or a glass of warm skim milk to help you doze off.

➤ Try to drink eight glasses of water a day to help flush out the system and relieve bloating.

➤ Exercise moderately at least three times a week. Walking and swimming are especially good for releasing stress and helping the cardiovascular system without adding the pounding pressure of high-impact aerobics.

➤ Take Tylenol or Advil to help with cramping, headache, and lower back pain.

➤ If you need a sugar "hit," try eating an orange. It's sweet, but prevents the hormone imbalancing effects of refined, processed sugar.

➤ Pepto-Bismol works for nausea. Also try a cup of herbal tea and plain toast. If your nausea is combined with headache, use Tylenol or buffered aspirin to avoid further stomach upset.

➤ Try vitamin and mineral supplements for mood swings. Calcium, a B-complex vitamin, and vitamins C and E may help.

Menstrual Cramps (Dysmenorrhea)

Yes, there really is a reason for menstrual cramping, and it has to do with hormones—specifically with the excess production of prostaglandins. These hormones, produced in the endometrium (the mucousy covering of the uterus), help the uterus contract, which is necessary for menstruation flow. Sometimes, however, these contractions hurt and cause cramps. Cramps can also be exacerbated if your body releases too much estrogen into the bloodstream. This increases fluid retention.

If you have dysmenorrhea, you are not alone. Approximately 50 percent of all women experience some degree of cramping during menstruation.

The best prevention for dysmenorrhea is the same for PMS: a salt-restricted diet, plenty of exercise, a good night's rest, and lots of water. A calcium-rich diet has also been found to help. Eat low-fat yogurt and drink skim milk or, if you "hate" dairy products, try a calcium-magnesium supplement. For minor cramps, an over-the-counter medication such as Midol can help. And if you can wear clothing that stretches around your waist and stomach, and can spend an hour resting with a heating pad for company, you might just find the cramps less severe.

> **First Things First**
> The best exercise for easing cramps is swimming. The water is soothing and cooling, and swimming is the least strenuous of all exercises. In addition, the endorphins (natural pain-killing hormones) released by your body during exercise, should help you get "in the swim" in no time!

If cramps interfere with your daily routine, see your physician. He or she can prescribe stronger medication to alleviate your pain.

Excessive Bleeding (Menorrhagia)

Every woman's definition of a heavy period is different. Some women *always* have a heavy flow during the first few days of menstruation and it's perfectly acceptable. Still others rarely have heavy bleeding.

Because it is so difficult to pinpoint when bleeding is too much, most physicians suggest this ground rule: if you need to change your tampon or sanitary napkin once or twice *every* hour, you have menorrhagia.

What causes excessive bleeding? Several things, ranging from the serious to those easily remedied:

Too much exercise or too strict a diet

Benign cysts in the uterus called fibroids

Urinary tract infection

Dysfunctional blood clotting

Perimenopause, or the very early stages of menopause

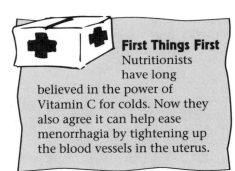

First Things First
Nutritionists have long believed in the power of Vitamin C for colds. Now they also agree it can help ease menorrhagia by tightening up the blood vessels in the uterus.

Although fibroids, infections, and clotting disorders need the attention of a physician, you can also help ease the flow by doing the following:

➤ Cut back on exercise

➤ Eat a more well-rounded diet

➤ Ease up on your workload to keep stress at a minimum

➤ Ask your doctor about iron supplements to keep energy up and prevent the possibility of anemia

Sporadic Bleeding

When spotting occurs is much more important than the fact that you do bleed on occasion. If the spotting occurs during ovulation, it is harmless. If your sporadic bleeding occurs around ovulation, even if it is accompanied by slight pain in the lower abdomen, you don't have to spend any sleepless nights full of worry (although you should check with your gynecologist just to be absolutely certain). However, if your sporadic bleeding occurs at any other time during your monthly cycle, it could signal something more serious, including:

Urinary tract infection

Endometriosis (inflammation of the uterine wall lining)

Benign fibroids in the uterus

Dysplasia (abnormal cell growth in the cervix)

Cervical cancer

Pregnancy problems

Hormonal imbalance (usually due to the wrong dosage of birth control pills)

First Aids
If you have been diagnosed with *dysplasia*, there's no need to panic. Abnormal cell growth usually doesn't mean cancer, and the questionable cells can be quickly removed in a doctor's office. But dysplasia *can* lead to cancer in some people—which makes an annual pap smear crucial.

If you have irregular spotting, it's important to see your gynecologist to rule out anything serious—and to take care of any problems before they get worse!

Before You Put the Band-Aid On

Endometriosis is an inflammation or an abnormal thickening of the mucous lining of the uterus. In most cases, endometriosis is asymptomatic; there are no symptoms. However, some women experience terrible period cramps. They might have pain on intercourse; their cycle might become irregular, spotty, or too heavy; they might have trouble getting pregnant. The good news is that the thick layers of endometriosis can be removed on an outpatient basis, using a laser process called a *laparoscopy*.

Skipping a Cycle

It sounds like a nightmare: PMS for two or three months with no relief in sight! Unfortunately, the stress of waiting for your period compounds the problem—because stress is one of the major culprits in irregularity. (Of course, pregnancy is still reason number one!) When stress strikes, unrelenting and from all directions, your brain sends out a message to the endocrine system: This is not a good time to get pregnant. The result? Your body might stop producing progesterone, a hormone necessary for ovulation, fertilization, and menstruation.

Of course, there are other reasons besides stress that can create hormonal imbalances that make you skip a cycle. They include:

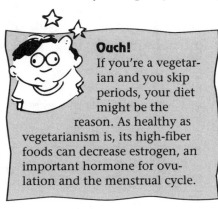

Ouch!
If you're a vegetarian and you skip periods, your diet might be the reason. As healthy as vegetarianism is, its high-fiber foods can decrease estrogen, an important hormone for ovulation and the menstrual cycle.

Too much high-impact, vigorous exercise

Adolescence (a teen's reproductive cycle has not completely matured)

Menopause

Yo-yo dieting (which wreaks havoc with your hormones)

Fibroids in the uterus

Endometriosis

Urinary tract infections (especially if accompanied by fever)

Cancer (in rare cases)

A woman's reproductive organs.

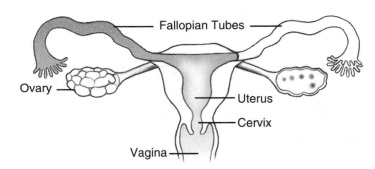

If you have an irregular cycle for more than three months, see your gynecologist. He or she can rule out any serious conditions or treat them before they get worse.

Emergency Tampons and Sanitary Napkins

There you are, out in the woods, enjoying your vacation to the max. The stress and the dull routines of your everyday life seem far, far away. But wait. There's one thing you didn't count on—your period. And you didn't bring any tampons or napkins. The first solution is an easy one. You can drive to a drug store and buy a box. However, if you're not near civilization or it's the middle of the night, this can be tricky. In emergency situations, practicality rules.

If you only have to wait until morning, use folded up tissue or toilet paper as a makeshift napkin. (After all, our grandmothers and their grandmothers used hand-washed rags that they frequently changed and cleaned. If they could do that, hey, what's a little inconvenience to us?)

If there's no chance of getting to a drugstore, supermarket, or convenience store, you can use thick wads of folded up paper towel or clean washcloths. In a real pinch, you can cut up a clean shirt or T-shirt into squares. Use two to three squares depending on your flow.

If you hate the idea of napkins, you'll just have to adjust. There's no safe way to make an emergency tampon. The probability of infection is just too high.

The Beastly Yeast Infection

The itchy, burning discomfort of a yeast infection is so common nowadays that over-the-counter medications are advertised on prime-time television. And, chances are, if you've had a yeast infection once, it will reoccur. Several factors give "rise" to yeast:

> **First Aids**
> The scientific name for a yeast infection is *Candida Albicans* or *Candida Monilia.*

> ➤ *Moist, dark, warm places.* You'll soon develop a full-fledged infection if you stay in a wet bathing suit all day, if you wear tight, constricted pantyhose and tights, and if you wear "unbreathable" latex or nylon panties. And talking about latex clothing, when you've finished an exercise session, it's important that you bathe and change to eliminate the sweat yeast thrives on.

> ➤ *A recent cycle of antibiotics.* Unfortunately, the medication you take to kill the "bad" bacteria also kills some of the "good" at the same time. This imbalance is just what yeast needs to grow.

> ➤ *Poor personal hygiene.* Besides warm locales, yeast also loves dirty places—the grimier the better.

> ➤ *Sexual intercourse.* Making love can transfer yeast infection from one partner to the other, ad infinitum, until it is cleared up in both of you.

> ➤ *Yeast allergies.* It's not something one wants to contemplate, but it is possible that your infection is caused by an allergic reaction to the yeast in foods. This means breads, pastas, pizza crusts, cakes, moldy cheeses, smoked meats, and more.

How Do You Know When You Have a Yeast Infection?

Let's put it this way. When you have a yeast infection, you'll know it immediately. The symptoms are hardly subtle. They include:

A terrible itch that just won't quit

Cottage cheese-like discharge

Burning during urination

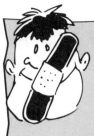

Before You Put the Band-Aid On

Although seven (long) days used to be the magic number when it came to yeast infections, you now can purchase over-the-counter three-day cures—and they work just as well. There's also a suppository you can use just one day, but it's only available by prescription. Check with your gynecologist.

To help relieve the symptoms of yeast infection while you're waiting for the medication to take effect, try soaking in a tub of warm water and baking soda. An oatmeal bath, such as Aveeno, will also soothe the itch.

The good news is that yeast infections are easily treated, especially today. Medications that used to be available only by prescription are now sold over-the-counter. These include Monostat 7 and Gynelotrimin, sold in seven-day doses of cream or suppositories. However, you should see your gynecologist before buying these products if you haven't had a yeast infection before; there's a chance your itching could be a sign of a different condition.

Also see your gynecologist if you have repeated yeast infections over a short period of time, such as three infections during the past three to six months. Recurrent infections can signal a serious condition or an underlying disorder, such as diabetes. Recurrent infections can also be an allergic reaction to either a contraceptive or even a partner. Whatever the reason, it's important to see your physician to determine what's going on.

Preventing the Beast Called Yeast

Yes, you can stop a yeast infection in its tracks before it begins. Here's how:

First Things First
The yogurts that work the best are 100 percent natural and have fresh, live *Lactobacillus acidophilus* cultures. You can find "blushing" fresh yogurt at health food stores and organic supermarkets.

➤ Wear cotton panties (or panties with cotton liners) that "breathe."

➤ Get out of your wet bathing suit as soon as possible.

➤ Eat a container of yogurt every day. (The active *Lactobacillus acidophilus* cultures found in yogurt keep yeast away.)

➤ Avoid refined sugar. (Sugar encourages the growth of yeast.)

➤ Stay away from feminine deodorant sprays, perfumed soaps, and scented oils. They can irritate the vaginal area—and put out a welcome mat to yeast.

If your infections keep coming back, see your doctor. It can signal a serious, underlying condition such as diabetes. If tests come back normal and you still get infections, consult an allergist. You might be allergic to yeast.

The Least You Need to Know

➤ Soothe breast tenderness with an ice pack or soft cotton inserted in your bra.

➤ Urinary tract infections (UTI) or cystitis won't go away by themselves. You need an antibiotic. You can help prevent UTI with cranberry juice or cranberry tablets.

➤ PMS is not "in your head." There are physiological reasons for everything from your mood swings to your bloating.

➤ Ease menstrual cramps with an easy, soothing exercise like swimming. Advil and Tylenol will also help ease cramps.

➤ Excessive bleeding is defined by having to change your tampon or sanitary napkin once or twice every hour.

➤ Yeast infections may be avoided by eating a container of yogurt every day. Many over-the-counter medications can successfully treat your yeast infection in three to seven days.

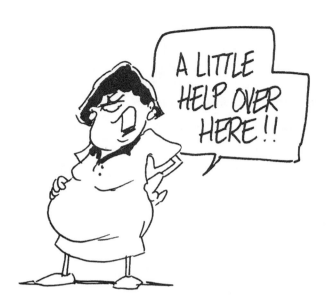

Chapter 29

Pregnancy Emergencies

In This Chapter

➤ Helping someone who is suffering from "morning sickness"

➤ Easing the discomfort of swollen ankles and minor cramps

➤ The signs of a *real* emergency—and the symptoms that are perfectly normal

Pregnancy is a time of joy. Mother Nature has been handling pregnancies since the beginning of humankind; a woman's body is designed, regulated, and adapted to ensure the health of a mother-to-be.

But, as we all know, complications can occur. Age, hormonal imbalance, infection, and various medical conditions can all interrupt Mother Nature's perfection. These complications can be as serious as a miscarriage—or as benign as early morning nausea.

When is a pregnancy emergency a real emergency, one that needs immediate medical attention? This chapter helps you make that decision.

The Mother-To-Be's Bane: Morning Sickness

It's as natural as a tiny toe's "thump" when you're lying in bed, as those "delightful" hemorrhoids that appear just when you think you can't take another indignity, as those cravings for pickles, ice cream, Big Macs, and shakes on a rainy, windy, miserable night. It's called morning sickness and it appears during the first trimester of pregnancy.

Here are some facts about the pregnant woman's version of getting nauseated and throwing up.

➤ Morning sickness can occur at any time during the day. Most woman get nauseous in the morning, but just because you might throw up at 9 o'clock at night, it doesn't mean there's anything wrong.

➤ If morning sickness continues after the third month, you should be checked out by your obstetrician as soon as possible.

➤ Morning sickness is a physical reaction to the extreme hormonal changes your body begins to go through during pregnancy.

There's not much you can do when Mother Nature decides to put a punch in your hormonal balance. It's a necessary and healthy component of pregnancy. But it would be nice if that "hormonal cocktail" didn't make you feel so nauseated—especially when, say, you're in the middle of a meeting or shopping at the mall.

Here are some tips that have helped other mothers-to-be. You might try them when morning sickness decides to wake up and do its thing:

➤ *Enjoy a breakfast in bed.* Eating some bland food, such as crackers or plain toast, can help prevent the worst of it.

➤ *Eat like a squirrel.* Nibbling all day long, instead of eating three square meals a day, will also help keep nausea at bay.

➤ *Try a Fruitopia.* If your nausea is accompanied by vomiting, you'll need to replace the fluids you lost. Fruit juices are especially good. They're full of vitamins and they contain carbohydrates—which help keep dehydration at bay. (Just ask any runner, pregnant or otherwise.)

Swollen Ankles: Another Delightful Side Effect

It's not that you're "fat." And it doesn't mean that your lower legs and ankles will always feel like they're the size of sump pumps. Swollen ankles during the last trimester are a normal part of many pregnancies.

What happens is that your abdomen, growing larger and larger to compensate for the almost-born baby in the uterus, presses on the vena cava (the main vein) that brings "used up" fluids back to the heart for an oxygen fix. The vein, reacting to this abdominal pressure, sends fluid down to the ankles and legs.

Here are some tips to help you combat puffiness:

➤ *Stay away from salt.* The more salt you eat, the more water you will retain, making swollen ankles worse.

➤ *Go out for a leisurely walk.* Walking is safe for pregnant women in the last trimester, provided you don't overdo. As you move, fluids pooled in your ankles will also move away from your ankles, circulating to other parts of your body.

➤ *Go for a swim.* Even if swimming wasn't such a great exercise because it helps to redistribute fluids and move muscles without energy, it would make you feel light and dainty— something every woman needs in the last few months. But swim slowly and don't overdo.

➤ *Keep your legs and feet elevated.* At night, while you're lying in bed, turn to the side, if possible, and keep your legs elevated with pillows. If you're watching TV on the couch, use a footstool to keep your legs up. This reduces pressure and moves pooled fluids back up.

> **Ouch!**
> It can be quite serious if swelling occurs in the arms and hands in the last trimester. This is a sign of *toxemia* and means that fluid retention is reaching dangerous levels. Other signs of toxemia include rapid weight gain, disorientation, blurry vision, terrible headaches, nausea, and decreased urination. If you experience any of these symptoms, immediately call for help to avoid the worst results of toxemia: convulsions and possible death.

Urinary Tract Infections: A Common Condition

The good seems to go hand-in-hand with the bad. The same reasons that make the uterus a perfect place for a fetus to grow—the warmth, the dark, the rich moisture—also make it a place where bacteria wants to congregate. This environment is one of the reasons why women are so susceptible to urinary tract infections. For more information on urinary tract infections see Chapter 28.

And, unfortunately, pregnant women are even more susceptible than their menstruating counterparts. The enlarging uterus bears pressure on so many organs, pushing down on the bladder, the kidneys, and the urethra. The irritation from this pressure combined with the hospitable environment makes a pregnant woman vulnerable to urinary tract infections (UTIs).

Although UTIs are not usually dangerous for pregnant women, they are more difficult to treat:

➤ Pregnant women should not take strong antibiotics, such as Septra (one of the most popular UTI medications).

➤ Because of the susceptibility in pregnant women, a UTI that finally dissipates is soon replaced by another.

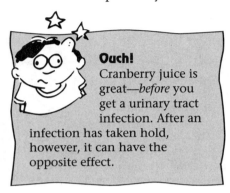

Ouch!
Cranberry juice is great—*before* you get a urinary tract infection. After an infection has taken hold, however, it can have the opposite effect.

The best solution? Live with it. But you don't have to be too stoic. There are some treatments that can help relieve the burning pain, including taking shallow, lukewarm sitz baths sprinkled with baking soda, urinating while standing in the shower, and practicing good personal hygiene.

There are also not-so-potent antibiotics that can be used to suppress the infection without increasing the risk of pregnancy complications. Ask your obstetrician about these if UTIs are a problem. (See Chapter 28 for a complete description of suggestions about UTI treatment.)

Signs of Dangerous Pregnancy Complications

Although the normal discomforts of pregnancy can be annoying, they are not life-threatening—and, when you're holding your new baby, who even remembers the swollen ankles, the UTIs, or the hemorrhoids! (See Chapter 27 for information on hemorrhoids.)

However, there are other symptoms that cannot be ignored and need attention immediately.

The Three Big Pregnancy "Tests"

There is nothing worse than the fear that something might be happening to your body when you are pregnant—something that might hurt your baby. The three most alarming warning signs that a pregnancy is at risk are spotting and bleeding, abdominal cramps, and sudden weakness.

Spotting can signal the onset of a miscarriage. Help the pregnant woman having these symptoms into bed. Have her rest completely, which means staying in bed. Call her obstetrician once she's settled in. Outright bleeding can be more serious, especially if clots or tissue are eliminated. A sudden heavy flow can signal a *spontaneous abortion* (which, in most cases, occurs when the fetus is deformed or problematic). Too much bleeding, however, can cause shock. Don't wait; get to the hospital as quickly as possible.

Mild abdominal cramps, even if accompanied by chills and fever, aren't necessarily a cause for alarm. Call the doctor and make the pregnant woman comfortable. Mild cramps can signal something as simple as slight pressure on the pelvic area. On the other hand, serious cramps are a different matter entirely. If they occur early in the pregnancy, the cramps can be a sign of an ectopic pregnancy. The cramps might also be accompanied by severe pain, nausea, chills, and fever.

> **First Aids**
> *Ectopic pregnancy* means that the fertilized egg never made it out of the fallopian tube and down to the uterus. Instead, the egg begins to grow and divide while it's in the small tube.

Today, an ectopic pregnancy can be corrected with an outpatient laser surgery. A tool called a laparoscope is inserted into the belly button while the patient is under anesthesia. If not treated and the egg continues to grow, the fallopian tube will eventually burst—and, like a ruptured appendix, infect the body. The end result can be shock, blood poisoning, and the loss of at least one fallopian tube.

> **First Aids**
> A *gynecologist* specializes treating conditions related to the female reproductive cycle. An *obstetrician* specializes in treating pregnant women. A *pediatrician* specializes in treating newborn babies, toddlers, and young teens.

Occurrences of sudden weakness can be the result of a sudden hormonal drop as the body adjusts to its pregnant state. If a pregnant woman experiences weakness that immediately passes, she need not do anything more than lie down for a while. However, it can't hurt to call the obstetrician, and definitely report anything out of the ordinary. On the more serious side, if the weakness is accompanied by signs of shock (such as rapid pulse, pale skin, chills, blurry vision, and irregular breathing), a woman should seek medical help immediately. (See Chapter 3 for a description of shock symptoms and treatment.)

While you are waiting for an ambulance to arrive, follow these guidelines for treating the pregnant woman:

> **First Things First**
> If a pregnant woman has been injured or is a victim of the flu or any other illness, call the doctor. Obstetricians are there to answer your questions, even if you think the questions sound bothersome. (In fact, if the physician does seem annoyed, get another one fast!)

➤ Position the pregnant woman on her left side.

➤ Make sure she is comfortable. Place a loose blanket around her.

➤ Keep the pregnant woman quiet and calm. Avoid making any sudden, jerky movements. Loud noises and bright lights can startle the woman and add to her stress.

The Least You Need to Know

➤ Thanks to Mother Nature, the fetus is normally secure and protected in the uterus. Diseases and accidents cannot easily penetrate the almost invincible womb.

➤ Be on the look-out for the "big three" warning signs of a serious problem: bleeding, abdominal cramps, and weakness.

➤ Call the obstetrician if a pregnant woman shows signs of anything out of the ordinary.

➤ Morning sickness, swollen ankles, and urinary tract infections are not usually dangerous, but call the doctor anyway.

➤ If a pregnant woman is spotting, get her into bed immediately. It can signal the onset of a miscarriage.

➤ Abdominal cramps that occur in the first months of pregnancy can signal an ectopic pregnancy.

➤ The worst case scenario when a pregnant woman experiences sudden weakness is that she will go into shock.

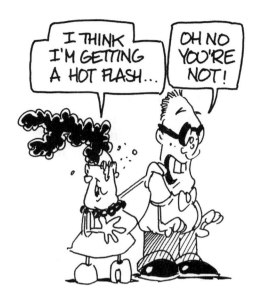

Menopausal Discomfort

Once upon a time, menopause was considered "the end" of youth and vitality. Women were suddenly old and "dried up." This belief was perpetuated by the fact that menopause was never discussed—and never, ever brought up in public.

All that has changed. Thanks to best-selling books, such as *The Silent Passage* by Gail Sheehy, magazine articles, and the ever-increasing number of women at menopausal age, menopause has "come out of the closet." It's talked about and discussed with as much openness as the latest movie or the latest office gossip.

Today, more is known about menopause than ever before. There are ways to treat its most distressing symptoms. And we know, without a doubt, that it doesn't have to "rob" us of anything. It's simply a biological occurrence, another chapter in the life cycle, and as natural as laughing, singing, and growing up.

Signs of Menopause

In scientific terms, menopause is a state in which the body's hormonal output of estrogen, a crucial component in pregnancy and menstruation, begins to decrease in irregular stops and starts. The body reacts, trying to readjust to this up and down pattern, causing the symptoms associated with menopause. Eventually, the estrogen regulates itself; the body adapts to the new, decreased level and the symptoms disappear.

But while these symptoms are in place, they can cause havoc in women. These symptoms are definitely not subtle:

Hot flashes	Memory loss
Depression	Loss of libido
Erratic mood swings	Fatigue
Irritability	Vaginal dryness
Water retention and weight gain	Increased vulnerability to yeast infections and cystitis

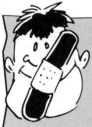

Before You Put the Band-Aid On

American women suffer more from menopausal symptoms than their Eastern neighbors. Japanese women have exceedingly fewer hot flashes; only about nine percent have any menopausal symptoms at all! This is due, in part, to their soy-rich diet. Soy is a food containing phytoestrogens that, when converted in the body, become estrogen.

Coping with the Big Four: Hot Flashes, Mood Swings, Depression, and Lack of Desire

Of all the symptoms associated with menopause, these four get the biggest complaints. They are the ones that can disrupt your life and interfere with your routine. They represent the "worst" of menopause, the symptoms that most have women running to their doctors for help.

Hot Flash! Hot Flash!

Approximately 85 percent of all American menopausal women suffer from hot flashes, those sudden,
intense, sweaty flushes that quickly turn into chills.
Most hot flashes occur in the middle of the night,
causing women to bolt up from a sound sleep. But
hot flashes can really happen at any time—in a
restaurant, during a meeting, or when you're in the
playground with your child.

Although hot flashes eventually pass once the body
adjusts to its new estrogen levels, they can be torture.
Here are some tips for welcome relief:

> **First Aids**
> *Perimenopause* is the
> medical term for the
> years leading up to
> menopause. During
> this time, estrogen is beginning
> its "push and pull," keeping you
> slightly off-balance. You can
> experience more intense PMS-
> like symptoms. You can start
> developing fibroids. Menstrua-
> tion might become heavier. (See
> Chapter 28 for more informa-
> tion.) You begin to experience
> the irritability and moodiness of
> menopause itself.

➤ *Do what the Japanese do: eat soy products.* Tofu,
   tempah, soy milk—all of these contain the
   phytoestrogens that create usable estrogen in
   the body.

➤ *Avoid caffeine.* The stimulant does just that—stimulating (or triggering) the body to
   raise blood pressure, create nervous tension, and add one or two of those hot flashes.

➤ *Try relaxing with deep breathing.* As soon as you wake up in the morning, during the
   afternoon, or in an evening yoga class, taking long, deep breaths and slowly exhaling will help steady your body and its out-of-kilter hormonal structure.

➤ *Fight hot with cold.* If you get a hot flash, be practical. Place a cool washcloth on your
   forehead. Wear loose clothing.

Before You Put the Band-Aid On

Sometimes those "whatchamacallit gadget" catalogues are right on target.
One of the novelties you can find in any hardware store, gadget shop, or
novelty catalogue is a miniature fan. Small enough to fit in your purse or your
desk drawer, this tiny fan whirls to life with two AA batteries. It's the perfect
antidote to afternoon hot flashes!

Swing High, Swing Low

Feeling exhilarated and energetic one minute, and then anxious, irritable, and hopeless the next? You've got 'em! They're called sudden mood swings, and they go hand in hand with the hormonal imbalance of menopause. The most important thing to do if you experience the intense highs and lows of mood swings is to recognize them for what they are: a symptom of menopause. There's no cause for panic; they will pass. In the meantime, try any of these suggestions for relief:

➤ *Fit routine exercise into your life*. It's good for the heart, the nerves, and the hormones.

➤ *Add calcium and magnesium to your diet*. (The calcium calms and the magnesium helps the body absorb the calcium.)

➤ *Listen to relaxation or visualization tapes*. Close your eyes, breathe deeply, and let your mind relax. Relaxation helps you gain back your self-control.

The Black Hole

Depression is a silent villain. It sneaks in and makes everything look bleak. You feel hopeless and helpless, hating your life—yet not able to do anything about your situation. And, as time goes by, the depression gets worse, spiraling you down into a place of inertia and insomnia. You lose the ability to enjoy life.

Physicians now agree that depression can be an organic illness, one that occurs because of hormonal changes or chemical deficiencies in the brain. The messages sent from nerve cell to nerve cell are subtly altered—for the worse. (See Chapter 16 for details on how the brain works.)

Antidepressant medications can help control the chemical imbalance, but because depression in menopause is linked closely to hormonal change, you might want to "wait it out."

➤ *Tell yourself this too shall pass*. Keep a note pasted on the bathroom mirror. Write in a journal. "Menopause will end—and with it my depression."

➤ *Pump up the exercise*. Vigorous exercise helps keep the blues away.

➤ *Establish a routine*. Get up at a certain hour every day and go to sleep at the same time every night. A routine helps regulate your body and gives you a sense of control.

➤ *Be good to yourself*. This doesn't mean bingeing on a bottle of booze and a double cheeseburger and fries. It does mean eating healthy foods and coping with stress in nondestructive ways. Take a bath with luxurious oils. Get a massage. Go for a manicure. Change your hair. And the noncaloric, nonalcoholic list goes on.

Some Like It Hot

We're not talking hot flashes here, we're talking sex. Unfortunately, the hormonal changes that occur in menopause can affect the libido. Suddenly, in otherwise healthy women, the sexual drive takes a drop. Add the fact of vaginal dryness and many women would just as soon curl up with a good book.

The good news is that loss of libido in menopause is only temporary. It goes away when menopause stops—and it sometimes comes back even stronger! But while you're waiting, try these suggestions for spicing up your love life:

➤ *Increase your appetite with erotica.* Try reading a poem, a novel, or whatever literature will help.

➤ *Add spice.* Try something new, be it a new technique or whatever. Use your imagination!

➤ *Lubricate.* There are many over-the counter creams on the market that can combat vaginal dryness. K-Y Jelly is one of them.

➤ *Take your time.* Don't feel pressured. Spend a sensuous hour in the bath. Plan a leisurely evening complete with candles and a wonderful meal. Let your partner help.

The Menopause Miracle: Hormone Replacement Therapy

Today, women have a choice. They don't have to "bite the bullet" and wait until menopause is over to ease its symptoms. Unlike previous generations, menopausal women now have hormone replacement therapy (HRT) which can combat the most intense problems of menopause: hot flashes, loss of libido, mood swings, and depression.

HRT must be prescribed by your physician. Only he or she can determine which is the best therapy for you. HRT is available in an estrogen only regimen and in a combination estrogen and progesterone regimen.

WARNING: Before we begin our discussion on the pros and cons of hormonal therapy, it's important to note that this is a highly controversial topic. The data physicians and scientists have gathered is inconclusive.

Estrogen Only (ERT): Pros and Cons

Estrogen comes in pills, skin patches, and vaginal creams (for dryness). Estrogen helps regulate your hormones, making you feel consistent and wonderful. It's not unusual for women to have a glow when they are on estrogen. Table 30.1 outlines the pros and cons of taking estrogen.

Table 30.1 Pros and Cons of Estrogen Only Therapy

Pros	Cons
Brings back sexual drive	Causes increased risk of uterine cancer
Causes hot flashes to disappear	May increase the risk of breast cancer in women with a history of breast cancer
Stops monthly "inconvenience" of menstruation. No more pads!	May increase susceptibility to osteoporosis (Regular exercise, such as walking, can help circumvent this risk.)
Ends depression	May cause recurrence in women who have previously been treated for breast cancer
Energizes the mind and body	
Regulates mood swings	
May reduce risk of heart attack	
Promotes a sense of well-being	

Before You Put the Band-Aid On

As a woman enters menopause, she is more at risk for osteoporosis. This can be counteracted by hormone therapy (a combination of estrogen and progesterone), by taking calcium-magnesium supplements (the magnesium helps the body absorb the calcium better), and through consistent exercise (such as walking). Although osteoporosis has been linked to genetic make-up, taking care of your body before menopause can halt some of the damage. This includes eating calcium-rich foods, taking calcium-magnesium supplements, and exercising—starting as early as possible!

If your physician decides that the risk of breast cancer and osteoporosis is too much, he or she might prescribe a *combination* of estrogen and progesterone.

Combination Hormone Therapy (HRT): Pros and Cons

A combination hormonal therapy more closely imitates a woman's natural cycle. Regimens vary slightly. An example is one in which the woman takes only estrogen on days 1–25. Then on days 16–25 progesterone is added. At the end of this cycle, the woman has a period. Table 30.2 weighs the pros and cons of HRT.

Table 30.2   Pros and Cons of Combination Hormone Therapy

Pros	Cons
Possibly decreases risk of uterine cancer	Sometimes causes intense PMS in second two weeks
Definitely decreases risk of osteoporosis	Monthly inconvenience of menstruation
Promotes a natural cycle	Progesterone may negate/nullify heart attack protection of estrogen
Offers a wonderful sense of well-being in first two weeks (due to the estrogen)	May cause recurrence in women who have previously been treated for breast cancer
Stops hot flashes	

*Studies conflict about the increased risk of breast cancer when on combination therapy.

The Least You Need to Know

➤ The four most common menopausal symptoms are hot flashes, mood swings, depression, and loss of libido.

➤ Hot flashes can be avoided naturally with soy products.

➤ Avoid mood swings with relaxation techniques.

➤ Fight depression with logical thinking and nondestructive rewards (such as tickets to a concert or a scented bath).

➤ HRT comes in two forms: estrogen only and an estrogen/progesterone combination. Estrogen only therapy offers a wonderful sense of well-being, but it may also increase the risk of uterine cancer. A combination regimen offers a more natural cycle.

➤ Each woman must be evaluated by a physician to determine which is the best regimen to try—if any.

Part 4
Sports and Travel First Aid

"There he is, he's running to first, passing second, it looks like a good one—oh no! He's down. Folks, he's down and he's not getting up..." Sports are wonderful to watch and participate in—as long as you realize that there are times you can get hurt. And, in today's world, where people are more athletic and fit than ever, there is a greater likelihood that an accident will occur because there are more people out there doing it!

And all the more reason you need to browse through the early chapters in this section. By the time you finish the chapter on jogging, swimming, and aerobic exercise, you'll be a one-person fighting first aid team!

On the other hand, maybe sports isn't your thing. Maybe it's travel. Well, when you travel to other areas, you encounter conditions that can cause very different types of medical emergencies than you might have to worry about at home. Don't worry. That's covered, too.

The Scouts have always said, "Be prepared." Well, that's just where this part comes in handy.

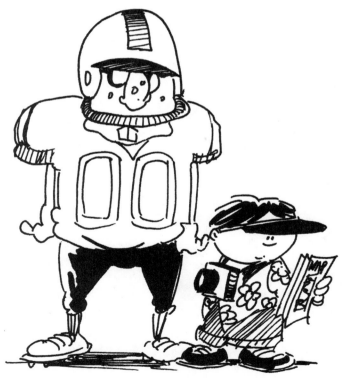

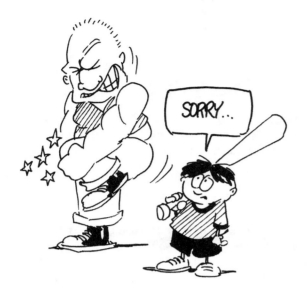

Chapter 31

Team Sports Injuries

In This Chapter

➤ Learn which sport has the most injuries—and why

➤ Discover what to do when an injury occurs on the playing field

➤ Find out how to make team sports practically injury-free

If you're an observer, sitting in the stands, watching a sport is a lot of fun. If you're a parent and it's your child out there hitting the ball, making the basket, or slapping the puck you'll be excited, but there will be a dose of terror mixed with that "fun."

The fact is that team sports, from hockey to football and from baseball to basketball, can be dangerous if proper precautions aren't met.

There are guidelines governing every sport. Officials and coaches should know them, but it doesn't hurt if you, too, understand the pitfalls of team sports. The state governments also have guidelines outlining specific safety rules for each sport. (For example, in New Jersey, if your child wants to play soccer on the school team, he or she must wear a helmet and shin guards. And many states require that only softballs are used in Little League games.) Your child might not be Michael Jordan, but he or she is still adored.

And, yes, you'd better believe it: Michael Jordan follows the guidelines of basketball very carefully! The penalty for not obeying the official rules can be as severe as suspension from a team.

Take Me Out to the Ball Game: Baseball

It's as American as apple pie and mom. It's the quintessential all-time American game, loved by everyone from eight-year-old Little League players to the parents playing on company teams. Baseball: nostalgic, beautifully orchestrated, and possibly hazardous to your health.

The Top 10 Baseball Injuries

Many children get their introduction to baseball in Little League or away at camp. You should make sure there is a capable coach supervising each camp—one who is not so enthusiastic that he asks kids to do dangerous things, such as leap too high for a fast ball, skid too fast into base, or throw the bat enthusiastically up into the air or out into the crowd where it can hit someone.

The baseball diamond's first aid kit should always include instant ice packs, adhesive bandages, sterile gauze pads, adhesive tape, scissors, first aid cream, rubbing alcohol, Ace bandages, and swatches of cloth to make slings for possible fractures and breaks.

Sprains, muscle pulls, broken bones, and concussions are the most common injuries. (For step-by-step instructions for first aid treatments of these conditions, see Chapters 21 and 16, respectively.) Specifically, you should be prepared for the following injuries:

➤ *Pitcher's elbow.* Baseball is a game with a lot of throwing action that puts pressure on the upper body. This condition, an inflammation of the bony joint of the elbow, occurs with repeated hard-slamming throws.

➤ *Leg sprains and breaks.* Baseball doesn't just involve the top part of an athlete's body. Every time a person throws a ball, the lower extremities get into the act. And don't forget those "sliding into base" moves.

➤ *Shoulder pull.* Another injury of the upper body, shoulder pulls occur from catching high balls, from throwing a ball to base with all you're worth or from hitting so hard with a bat, it cracks.

➤ *Concussion.* Even softballs can pack a wallop when they're thrown at top strength. Unfortunately, baseball players don't wear headgear (caps don't count), and sometimes baseballs land where they shouldn't ...on vulnerable heads.

➤ *Cracked teeth.* Baseball players don't wear mouthguards either, and the ball that misses the top of the head can get the teeth.

➤ *Broken jaw.* The jaw, too, is exposed to flying baseballs during a game. A ball might hit a child on the outside of the jaw or face forward. Even a mouthguard can't protect against that.

➤ *Black eye.* By now, you know the culprit, a hard thrown ball. But, sometimes, a baseball bat can be the culprit. Maybe an enthusiastic hitter, running off to first, throws his bat—and, unfortunately, it lands on your child, who just happens to be sitting in the bleachers or waiting for his turn at bat.

➤ *Heat Prostration.* When an inning lasts forever in the hot sun, the pitcher can begin to look like Gatorade.

➤ *Foot Injury.* Sneakers are not always the best shoe to protect toes from getting stubbed or broken. Making a run to a base or getting hit in the foot from a bat or a ball is all it takes.

➤ *Back Injury.* Picking up foul balls, bending to catch a low-flying ball, jumping at an angle to get a curving ball—all of these cause back injury.

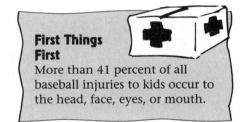

First Things First
More than 41 percent of all baseball injuries to kids occur to the head, face, eyes, or mouth.

Treatment and Prevention

Flexibility is key for back and shoulder injuries, sprains and breaks. All it takes is a warm-up before a game, plus five minutes of stretches, to keep muscles and joints limber, supple, and resilient.

Most fitness and exercise books offer good stretching exercises, providing both step-by-step instructions and illustrations. Some of our favorites include *The Rockport Walking Program* by James Rippe, M.D. and Ann Ward, with Karla Dougherty (published by Fireside Books) and *Aerobics* by Kenneth Cooper (published by Bantam Books). Your local Y should have drawings of stretches clipped on a bulletin board. And the President's National Council on Fitness, based in Washington, D.C., also has information on the best stretches to perform before exercising.

Although headgear and mouthguards are only found on umpires and the occasional pitcher, all players would do well to arm themselves with this protection. It would stop many tragic accidents to the head, face, eyes, and mouth.

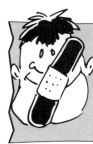

Before You Put the Band-Aid On

The best warm-up for any exercise is the exercise you are about to do—but at a slower pace. Walk around the playing field, gently "hit" the air with a bat or racquet, or play a leisurely game of catch with a teammate.

Hoop Dreams: Basketball

Basketball is taking the country by storm. It's becoming the number one game in America according to experts (those who love basketball!) In fact, tickets are so hot for professional and collegiate basketball games, that fans will pay more than $1,000 for one ticket!

The 10 Top Basketball Injuries

Basketball can also be fraught with injury if the game isn't closely supervised by a referee who is vigilant in calling fouls. Most team players have to watch out for getting kicked and shoved by players on the other team. You can have a bad fall, pulling muscles and breaking bones, if you are pushed to the floor.

The basketball team's first aid kit should include adhesive bandages, ice packs, pain relievers, instant ice bags, adhesive tape, scissors, sterile gauze pads, first aid cream, Ace bandages, and swatches of cloth for making slings. For step-by-step first aid treatment for specific injuries, see the appropriate chapter in Part 2.

➤ *Shoulder injury.* Hurtling basketballs into the basket over and over again can cause an arm or shoulder to get out of joint.

➤ *Tendonitis.* All that jumping, scooping, and bending can be hard on muscles, especially those in the lower calf. The painful condition known as tendonitis can result; it is an inflammation of the tendons that connect the leg muscle to the bone.

➤ *Bursitis.* Guard duty can be fun, but it puts a lot of stress on the ankles—leading to bursitis. This is a painful swelling of the *bursa*, the sac-filled cushion at the heel. This same condition can affect the bursa in the shoulder and elbows, which is often felt by centers, for example, who keep their arms up in the air for long periods of time.

➤ *Impingement Syndrome.* When shoulders are overused, calcium deposits will some-times settle in the ligaments that connect the collarbone with the shoulder blade. Deposits can also accumulate in the hips, knees, ankles, wrists, and even the fingers. The result? Every time a player reaches for the basket, it hurts!

➤ *Lower back pain.* Repetitive bending, as in guarding the other team's best player, can hurt even the youngest backs.

➤ *Carpal tunnel syndrome.* Dribbling heavy, bouncing balls might earn you a basket, but it can also cause carpal tunnel syndrome, a condition in which the ligament band that goes around nerves and muscles that runs from the fingers through the arm, is constricted. Nerves literally "hit" muscle and bone, causing excruciating pain.

➤ *Jumper's knee.* Even if you are light on your feet, all that jumping can eventually take its toll—causing swelling and inflammation. That's why so many professional basketball players wear Ace bandages, more constrictive wraps, or even braces on their knees when they're on the court.

➤ *Foot injury.* Think of it. All that movement, feet jumping, balls bouncing, arms waving, your eye's on the ball and ouch! It's not uncommon for one player to fall and turn an ankle or for someone to unintentionally step on the toe of another player.

➤ *Neck pain.* Shoulders and arms do a lot of the work, but the neck also gets into the act. Throwing that ball up, pushing it through a basket, looking up, these actions curl the neck into uncomfortable, strenuous positions.

➤ *Eye injuries.* According the National Basketball Association, black eyes, cuts and scrapes around the eye, and bruises in the area of the eye are among the most common injuries in the sport. Many players are sidelined by eye injuries, unable to play because their eyes are swollen shut and bandaged, or because their sight is impaired.

Treatment and Cures

As in any team sports, flexibility is key. Keeping muscles supple and loose is vital for keeping strains and sprains to a minimum. Basketball players should concentrate on the upper body, especially the arms, neck, and shoulders, performing at-home stretches and strengthening these muscles on gym machines in-between games.

Knees, too, are problem areas in basketball. The best treatment here is exercise, specifically leg lifts and machines that strengthen the knee's supporting muscles. Wearing an Ace bandage on an already sore knee can help prevent it from getting worse, but unless you're a pro, you're best off staying off the court until it heals.

20 Yards, 10 Yards, Touchdown!: Football

Ah, autumn. The brilliant leaves, the cool, crisp air, the cheering, screaming sounds coming from the stadium. Yes, it's football season, and already everyone's counting the days until the Super Bowl. Football is an American tradition, but all that sweat and glory can leave a host of injuries in its wake.

The 10 Top Football Injuries

There are more guidelines governing this sport than any other because the potential for injury is so great. Tackles, punches, and falls can all lead to sprains, breaks, and concussions. Broken noses are also a common problem. Despite the fact that players are required to wear protective gear, the game can become intense. And sometimes, for example, that headgear that's worn for protection, can be shoved up and cause even more damage! There's a reason why moms of teenage boys get nervous when their sons make the team!

First aid kits should include bandages, adhesive tape, scissors, first aid ointment, pain killers, rubbing alcohol, sterile eye wash, and instant ice packs. For step-by-step first aid treatment, see the chapters in Part 1 for treating emergencies or the chapters in Part 2 for treating specific injuries.

➤ *Cervical spine injury.* The violent, high-velocity impact that makes fans cheer is the same one that causes back and spinal cord injury. Just ask anyone who's ever had six players jump on top of him and the football.

➤ *Neck injury.* Quarterbacks are always craning their necks as they hop from one obstacle to another in the race for the goal, not to mention that fast-moving, fast-driving impact when they are tackled.

➤ *Knee injury.* Running, jumping, tackling …all of these moves put a great deal of pressure on the knee, causing it to swell or become dislocated.

➤ *Broken nose.* Some veteran football pros say you're not a seasoned player until you've had your nose broken—at least once. Although headgear has helped decrease the incidence of broken noses, six big guys on top of another guy (whose head is in the dirt) can make the protection worthless.

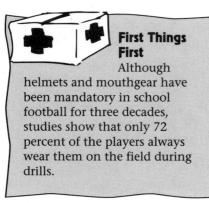

First Things First
Although helmets and mouthgear have been mandatory in school football for three decades, studies show that only 72 percent of the players always wear them on the field during drills.

➤ *Head injury.* Helmets are mandatory for football players, but, sometimes, in the heat of a tackle, the helmet can be dislodged. And, other times, a hard tackle from the back of the knees brings the player down—fast and hard—on his head. The helmet prevents some injury here, but not all of it.

➤ *Black eye.* Football can be a violent game. Witness the incidence of black eyes among players. A thrown football, an accidental tackle that lands a hand or foot above the face guard, even a knock on a helmeted head, can all cause a black eye.

➤ *Tendonitis*. The painful inflammation of the Achilles' heel (or tendon), the tendon that runs from the ankle to the heel, is common in football. Which isn't surprising when you think of the running, pounding, and tackling that takes place during the game.

➤ *Sprains and breaks*. It's obvious where these come into play—even with shoulder pads, mouthgear, and helmets. Tackles, falls, pushes, and grabs—the basics of football—can all result sprains or breaks.

➤ *Shoulder injury*. Reaching for a thrown football, straining to reach the goal with the ball grasped in your hand, stretching your arms while flat on the ground…these are movements that can cause shoulder injury.

➤ *Broken teeth*. Even if a player is wearing a protective mouthguard, teeth can be pushed in, broken, and chipped if the face hits the ground with force (or if those six guys once again jump on top of you and the football).

First Aids
The Achilles' Heel is named for a Greek warrior named Achilles, a man of such strength that he could never be beaten. His only vulnerable spot on his invincible body was the tendon that ran from the back of his ankle to his heel.

Before You Put the Band-Aid On

In football, a stubbed toe is called a "turf toe." It occurs when a player kicks the football over and over again or when a player's foot is pushed into the ground (sort of like being up on toeshoes without the shoes), and it can cause painful swelling, sprains, and even broken toes. The worst part of "turf toe" is the fact that the player has to be off his feet until it clears up (anywhere from two weeks to a whole season). Running and walking, especially in football shoes, is particularly painful.

Treatment and Cures

Once again, the name of the game is flexibility. Strength-training exercises on gym machines will help vulnerable knees, legs, shoulders, backs, and necks. Warm up jogs around the stadium are mandatory, as are stretching exercises before the game begins.

And even more important: wear your gear. The helmet and the mouthgear won't help if they're in your locker!

Last, but certainly not least, make sure your child's coach goes over proper tackling techniques over and over again. Teammates should know how to tackle safely. Many neck injuries result from a move called "spearing," in which a player tackles by attacking helmet-first instead of with the body.

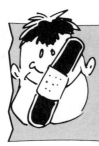

Before You Put the Band-Aid On

For foot and ankle pain, think of RICE: Rest, Ice, Compression, and Elevation. If you can get off the field, do so! Implementing these four measures will decrease swelling, pain, and inflammation.

The Iceman Cometh: Hockey

Think of your favorite football player in ice skates, and you get the image of what hockey is all about. But it goes three steps better when it comes to injury:

1. Ice is harder than dirt.

2. Skates have sharp blades.

3. Hockey sticks make better weapons than footballs do.

The 10 Top Hockey Injuries

Not every high school has a hockey team. They are mostly found in the colder regions of the country. But that doesn't mean that ice hockey is any less dangerous. Think of it as football—with the added danger of playing on ice. No wonder mothers and fathers contemplate moving to Florida! Beware the overzealous coach who dares players to improperly tackle and kick.

Common injuries include concussions and breaks resulting from falls on hard ice, and cuts from sharp skate blades. Players can also get frostbite. A first aid kit should include pain killers, adhesive bandages, sterile gauze pads, waterproof adhesive tape, rubbing alcohol, first aid cream, and insulated blankets.

For step-by-step first aid treatment, see Chapters 3 and 4 for treating such emergencies as bleeding, bandaging cuts and wounds, immobilizing, and treating for shock. See Chapter 11 for ear, eye, and nose damage, Chapter 8 for bumps and bruises, Chapter 16 for head injury, Chapter 20 for mouth and teeth injury, and Chapter 21 for sprains and breaks.

➤ *Lower back problems.* Hockey players are always bending, looking down at the puck, aiming, and hitting. This constant bending motion can create aches and pains in the lower back area.

Before You Put the Band Aid On

Athletes learn early on whether they are "loose-jointed" or "tight-jointed." For players who are hyperflexible and loose, flexibility isn't a problem. Strength is. They need to concentrate on strength-training exercises, using weights and gym machines. "Tight-jointed" players, on the other hand, have strong, tense muscles, ones that pull and strain. These athletes must stretch every day to gain flexibility.

➤ *Neck injury.* The same bending motion that affects the lower back can also strain the upper back and neck as well. Add turning your head to aim while bending and you have the makings of an injury.

➤ *Foot injury.* You won't see too many hockey players with flat feet, but, even so, skating for hours at a time can cause havoc to toes, heels, and ankles. The lack of circulation, the unrelenting pressure on the heel, the tight lacings at the ankle—all of these can cause problems.

➤ *Tendonitis.* Hockey players are vulnerable to the painful inflammation of the tendon at the back of the leg. Why? All that skating combined with the twisting and turning of the game adds unrelenting pressure to the leg.

➤ *Head injury.* Ice is slippery, and more than one hockey player has had his helmet skid off when he was checked and fell down hard.

➤ *Black eye.* Hockey players are required to wear helmets, headgear, shoulder pads, and knee pads. But only the goalies get a special head "cage" to protect their faces. A misaligned hockey stick or a high-stepping puck can use vulnerable eyes as a target.

➤ *Broken teeth.* Remember the rule: ice is harder than dirt. Even with protective gear, teeth can chip, break, and splinter if a player falls down hard.

➤ *Frostbite.* If the bleachers are cold, you can imagine how cold the actual arena is. Hockey players might build up a sweat as they race across the ice, but their hands are always grasping their hockey stick and their feet are immobile in their skates. This lack of movement interferes with circulation. Gloved hands, sock-covered feet, and even masked faces can feel this painful effect of the unrelenting icy cold when it lasts for longer than 20 minutes.

➤ *Cuts and bleeding.* Ice hockey has the added dimension of skates—with razor sharp blades. Fast, faster, faster still, the other team charges, sliding along on their skates. One player checks you, then another. Another falls—and cuts your arm with the bottom of his blade.

➤ *Spinal cord injury.* Sometimes the whole back is involved in a fall. Ice is slippery, and players will fall. Some of them fall backward, right on their backs. If a player injures his spinal cord, he might not be able to move. As in football, head, neck, and back injuries can occur with poor technique. Checking, ice hockey's version of tackling, must be taught and rehearsed over and over again to help reduce injury.

➤ *Broken bones.* Even with the use of shoulder pads, shin guards, and other gear, bones can get broken. A player might look like a superpower hero from Star Wars, but one bad check to the boards, and a twist or an awkward fall can bypass protection and cause a break.

On Thin Ice: Treatment and Cures

Backs can become stronger if players concentrate on strengthening their thighs and posterior muscles. By making these muscles strong and flexible, they can act as a "pedestal" for the bent back, preventing strain.

Hockey players need frequent breaks to avoid frostbite and other circulatory problems. Before playing hockey it is a good idea to add dollops of petroleum jelly on your lips, wear layers under your uniform and flex your hands frequently on the ice.

And, as always, don't forget your ice-skating warm up and those all important stretches on the inside bar of the arena.

Sock It to Me: Soccer

Once upon a time, soccer was *the* game only in Europe and South America, a tradition as strong as baseball in America. But it's only recently that soccer as a professional team sport has gained respect here as well.

But as a team sport for children, soccer has been just as popular here as abroad for years. Pass any suburban school yard, today or 20 years ago, and there are children, kicking a ball and trying to score a goal first.

There's a reason for soccer's popularity in the school yard. Of all the team sports, soccer is believed to be the least hazardous to a person's health. But, as with anything to do with kicking or moving fast, there are a few dangers attached. And, as the number of children playing the sport increases, so does the number of serious injuries.

The Soccer Injury Countdown

Most schools have extensive guidelines on soccer safety rules. Parents should receive a printed guide, listing the equipment they'll need for their children (such as shin guards, soccer shoes, and helmets) and safety measures that must be taken. Coaches should be on the field at all times, watching for potential problems with a diligent eye.

First aid kits for soccer should include adhesive bandages, sterile gauze pads, rubbing alcohol, instant ice packs, Tylenol, and first aid cream. For step-by-step information on first aid treatment for specific injuries, refer to the appropriate chapter in Part 2.

➤ *Ankle injury.* The very nature of soccer's method of kicking, with an awkward instep motion, makes players vulnerable to sprains and breaks to ankle bones.

➤ *Cuts and bruises.* Soccer is very animated at times, with lots of kicking. This can result in a fall or two—which, in turn, results in those ubiquitous knees and arms that get cut on rocks or the hard dirt of the playing field. Children can also get spiked by another player's shoe.

➤ *Black eyes.* A ball can sometimes fall short of its goal—and hit an unsuspecting player.

➤ *Back problems.* During intense periods of running up and down the playing field, a player can fall—and, like dominoes, six other guys can fall on top of him. The heavier the group, the heavier the pressure on the first player who fell. Tackling is allowed in soccer, but as in ice hockey and football, technique must be taught and rehearsed over and over again to avoid injury to all players.

Treatment and Cures

Years ago, children used to play soccer in sneakers and shorts—which could lead to some of the injuries discussed here. Today official rules and regulations make the game even safer. All players must wear shin guards and special soccer shoes. Helmets are required in some states. Hopefully, they will become law throughout the country to avoid possible head injury.

Flexibility and leg-strengthening exercises are just as important in soccer as they are in any sport. And don't forget to warm up and stretch (even if you're just chasing your little brother around the field).

The Least You Need to Know

➤ Baseball is the number one favorite game in American schools.

➤ Pitcher's arm is a baseball injury that is caused by an inflammation of the elbow and arm muscles.

➤ Basketball's most dangerous injuries involve the upper body.

➤ Football and hockey injuries, even with helmets and other safeguards, can be among the worst, including head injuries and spinal cord problems.

➤ Soccer is currently the safest team sport when it comes to severe neck and back injuries. But please note: the number of knee injuries, sprains, and broken bones have increased because more children are playing soccer in school.

➤ Always warm up and stretch before any sport.

➤ Flexibility and strength-training exercises are vital in preventing injury to muscles and joints.

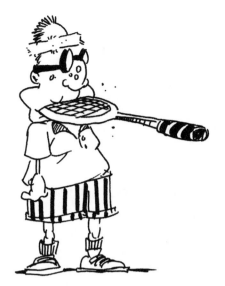

Chapter 32

Injuries in Individual Competitions: Golf, Tennis, and Skating

In This Chapter

➤ The most common golf injury

➤ How extreme temperatures can affect your golf game

➤ How "tennis elbow" got its name

➤ The joys—and the dangers—of inline skating

➤ Exploring ways to avoid ice skating injury

Ah, the perfect whoosh of a golf ball sailing in the air …the swing of a racquet …the wind whistling past your skates. One-on-one competition has its own joys and its own rewards. From tennis to golf, these types of sports enhance concentration. They teach you balance and focus. They also help people cope with stress in ways that are *good* for the body.

One-on-one recreational or competitive sports are a wonderful way to spend your leisure time. They are healthy; they reduce stress; they're a great excuse to get outside!

But, along with all these positives, there are a few negatives. Medical emergencies are the most important of these negatives—and the most dangerous. This chapter shows you how to cope with situations that occur when you're enjoying your favorite form of recreation.

To a Tee: Golf Injuries

Golf satisfies many needs all at once: the need for peaceful surroundings, the need for quiet, the need to, well, whack a golf ball and feel the vibrations as it sails up and over, landing directly on the green. Satisfaction? There's nothing like it for many.

But that little ball and that frail-looking metal club can cause a bit of havoc if you're not careful.

Watch Out for the Misguided Golf Ball

If you're Arnold Palmer, chances are you're not going to hit that small, hard ball into the crowd. But, beginners and advanced players alike will sometimes go where others "fear to tread." Maybe you're just learning how to hit the ball. Maybe your calculations are a fraction off. Maybe you've been stung by a bee just as you struck the ball. Whatever the excuse, a misguided golf ball can be dangerous. It can hit someone at a velocity that can cause brain damage if it goes to the head, or a dislocated shoulder or broken ankle if it hits the upper torso or the lower leg.

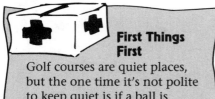

First Things First

Golf courses are quiet places, but the one time it's not polite to keep quiet is if a ball is moving right at another person. A general rule of etiquette and safety is to not tee off until all other golfers are out of the way.

The best element in this situation is a strong pair of lungs—or a whistle. Shout as quickly and as loudly as you can: "FORE!" (which in golf talk means "Ball coming!") if the ball in question is sailing toward another person.

If someone is hit, see if any damage has been done. Be prepared to get help immediately if necessary. See Chapter 16 on head injury and Chapter 21 on sprains and breaks for step-by-step first aid treatment for those particular injuries.

Arm and Shoulder Cramps

When you repeatedly swing a golf club, the tendons in your shoulders can become inflamed and swollen. They rub against the bone again and again. The result is painful cramps and tendonitis. (See Chapter 31 for treatment of tendonitis.)

Bursitis, another shoulder inflammation, is also caused by repetitive motion. But it comes with a not-so-special bonus: swelling in the bursa, the soft fluid-filled cushions found in the joints of the shoulder, elbow, or hip.

Dislocation is actually as it sounds. As you swing the club, your shoulder can move out of its socket—causing terrible pain.

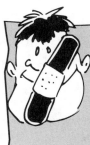

Before You Put the Band-Aid On

Never try to pop a shoulder back by yourself. It can cause even more damage—not to mention pain—if it moves. Your best bet is to quickly get the person to the emergency ward, after applying a loose wrap to keep the injured shoulder from "jostling." Signs of dislocation include:

Awkward position of limb

Intense pain at dislocated point

Pale, clammy skin

Only a physician can help a bad cramp or "pop" a dislocated shoulder back, but there are things you can do to ease the pain before you reach the emergency ward:

➤ Apply ice to the shoulder or arm immediately to reduce swelling. Ice the area several times a day for 15 to 20 minutes.

➤ Rest. Do not try to play another round of golf.

➤ If the pain still persists after three days, change to a moist heating pad. This increases circulation and keeps the area flushed with blood.

➤ Hot showers help soothe the pain.

When the pain is gone, increase your arm and shoulder endurance with stretching exercises. (See Chapter 31 for a full description of specific exercises.)

Leg Cramps and Soreness

Shin splint is a "catch-all" term used to describe any tendonitis, soreness, or cramp in the leg. But whatever its name, the reason for tendonitis, soreness, and cramping are always the same: overuse and misuse—which cause irritation and inflammation of muscle tissue.

Leg cramps and muscle soreness in golf can be the result of:

➤ A badly fitting pair of shoes

➤ Standing on your feet too long

➤ Too zealous a turn on the swing

The best treatment is RICE: Rest, Ice, Compression, and Elevation. Leg-strengthening exercises and stretches also help. Always warm up by walking around a part of the course before beginning your golf game.

Under Par: Extreme Temperature Conditions

Playing golf is wonderful exercise, especially for older adults. The scenery, too, is beautiful; golf courses are often in tropical climes or only open in the spring and summer. This, too, can be a good thing—unless the weather is particularly hot.

If you're out on the fairway in the blazing sun and suddenly feel…

Hot and cold at the same time

Chilled and sweaty at the same time

Faint and dizzy

Breathless

…you could be suffering from heatstroke or heat prostration (also called heat exhaustion). Have your golf partner get help as soon as possible. While you are waiting, get under the shade of a tree. Sip water, and loosen your clothes. Check for irregularities in breathing or pulse. (See Chapter 18 for a full description of heat prostration and how to treat it. See Chapter 3 for treatment of shock.)

Lightning Bug

Another common—and scary—golfing hazard is being hit by lightning. Suppose you are on a beautiful course, enjoying the beauty of the trees and your golf game, when boom! A sudden summer storm hits. Because you are surrounded by trees, you are a prime candidate for being hit by lightning.

This usually sounds more hazardous than it seems. Many people who get hit by lightning feel a sudden jolt and then nothing. They don't remember the incident, but they have no other side effects.

If someone you know is hit by lightning, make sure that he or she...

➤ goes directly to the emergency ward to make sure there has been no further damage to the body.

➤ lies prone.

➤ remains warm. (Cover him or her with a loose blanket if necessary.)

➤ is being watched for shock and the ABCs of first aid care: Airways clear, Breathing normal, Circulation fine.

> **First Things First**
> Did you know that in the 19th century golf balls were made of leather stuffed with feathers? The balls might not have traveled as far, but they sure caused fewer head injuries!

Follow the first aid treatments outlined in Chapter 3 for shock and in Chapter 8 for burns and electrical shocks.

"Tennis, Anyone?" Injuries on the Court

Some people need their tennis the way other people need their favorite chair. It just makes them feel good. They'll join clubs, go to resorts with courts, or, if they're really lucky, they'll put courts in their backyards.

Whether your idea of racquet heaven is tennis, squash, or racquetball, you'll understand this feeling. The exhilaration as ball meets racquet and you swing, the intense focus in which everything else drops away—you wouldn't give it up for the world.

But tennis does have its own "set" of injuries. If you don't treat them properly, it's possible you'll have to hang up your racquet—at least for a while.

Racquet or Tennis Ball Hits

It's bad form to throw your racquet at your opponent if you've lost the game. But accidents will happen and, occasionally, instead of a handshake, you'll get a racquet sailing across the net! More common is the tennis *ball*, which sometimes has a mind of its own. Sometimes, it goes right for your head instead of the center of your racquet.

A tennis ball or racquet going at full speed is no laughing matter. If it hits your head or your stomach, it can cause damage. The best medicine is prevention. Duck! (And consider getting rid of your tennis partner!)

If a hit is inevitable, call for help immediately. Treat the condition as you would any first aid emergency for cuts, bruises, or head injuries. (See Chapter 3 for information on treating wounds and cuts, Chapter 8 for bumps and bruises, and Chapter 16 for head injuries.)

Achilles' Folly

Tendonitis is one of the most common tennis ailments. Tendonitis is inflammation of the tendons that connect muscle to bone, including the one that reaches from the ankle to the heel (known as the Achilles' tendon).

The reason for irritated tendons is misuse. Maybe you pound the court with your feet as you hit the ball. Or maybe you try to get a shot that's a long leap—literally. Or perhaps you've tried to play too hard too soon. Whatever the reason, leg pain isn't going to go away unless you get off the court as soon as you feel the first pang of pain.

Remember RICE: Rest, Ice, Compression, and Elevation? It works here, too. And don't forget to take Tylenol, ibuprofen, or extra-strength aspirin to relieve the pain!

Although it's difficult to heal, you should cut down on the tennis until you are less "tender" and more "heeled." It could mean the difference between getting back on the court soon—or never.

Here are some hints to prevent leg pain:

➤ Strengthen abdominal muscles. If you do sit-ups or stomach crunches every day, your strong stomach will relieve some pressure from your lower back and legs.

➤ Make your leg muscles more flexible with stretching exercises.

➤ Warm up on a treadmill or a walk around the club. Warm muscles are less likely to tighten up and become injured.

➤ Lose weight. Excess pounds put pressure on legs—and slow down your tennis game.

First Things First

Camp used to be just for kids. No more. Today's tennis camps and clinics can teach you proper technique during one-on-one sessions and in small groups. You'll leave with more than improved scores—your safety skills will be intact. And you should have a great time, too! For a listing of good tennis clinics, call the National Tennis Association.

The Condition That Has Its Own Brand Name: Tennis Elbow

Actually, tennis elbow can happen in any sport that involves repetitive arm movement. It can even happen to carpenters who hammer all day long. Tennis elbow is an inflammation around the bony knob on the outside of the elbow and the surrounding area. It often occurs in tennis players when shock absorption is poor on serves and backhand strokes.

The best first aid care for tennis elbow is prevention. Here are some tips to keep tennis elbow from interfering with your game:

➤ Keep up with the latest news in tennis magazines, at your club, and during games on TV. New serving and stroke techniques are always being introduced after careful bioengineering tests at sports equipment companies.

➤ A new racquet might prove to be better in absorbing shock if it's not strung as tightly. This way the racquet, not your arm, absorbs the shock.

➤ Elastic bands and splints can change the point of tension in the arm, moving it away from vulnerable elbows and wrists.

➤ Hand and arm flexibility exercises can help make injured limbs stronger and keep healthy limbs flexible and loose.

Dehydration and Heatstroke

If you play tennis in an air-conditioned club, you won't suffer from extreme temperatures. But, if you love to play outside, there are some steps you should take to avoid heat prostration and dehydration:

➤ *Wear white.* There's a reason why tennis players wear white—and it has nothing to do with chic. White deflects the heat of the sun, keeping you cool inside.

➤ *Avoid the noonday sun.* For the same reasons it's best not to be on the beach in the scorching noon hours, tennis is a game that should be played in the early morning or the early evening. No one needs the sun's harmful rays beating down while he's trying to hit a ball.

➤ *Keep a water bottle nearby and use it during frequent breaks.* The more water you drink the better. Before the next serve or whenever you feel thirsty, call a break and head for the water bottle.

If you feel any of the symptoms of heat prostration (see Chapter 18), call for help immediately.

On Thin Ice: Skating Injuries

Skaters either glide over ice in colorful costumes or head for the concrete hills in colorful inline skates. Either way, skating is a lot of fun. Of all the individual competitive sports, skating is the most dangerous. Although there are fewer sprains and strains, broken bones are more common.

But, if you know what you're doing, there's nothing quite like the joy of spinning down a road or shimmering over cold ice, turning and dipping and seeing the sights go by. Whether rushing down a city sidewalk or gliding over cold ice, both forms of skating require instruction.

315

Inline Skating

Children as young as five are taking to the streets, skating past their elders with the speed of a greyhound. This, of course, can make for an occasional injury: broken bones, sprained wrists, bruised knees, and concussions. But if a child wears the proper safety equipment, why shouldn't he or she enjoy the fastest growing recreational sport in America? Proper equipment *always* includes wrist guards, knee pads, elbow pads, and a helmet.

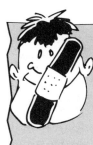

Before You Put the Band-Aid On

A study printed in a recent *Journal of the American Medical Association* reports that 30,000 injuries a year are caused by inline skating. And, as the sport continues to grow in popularity, the number of injuries will increase proportionately.

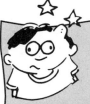

Ouch!

It's inevitable that at least once while you're skating, you're going to fall. Here's the best way to avoid injury during a fall:

1. As you fall, roll with it.

2. Avoid the instinct to catch yourself with your arms.

The best bet is to practice falling at home, in the privacy of your living room or bedroom. Carpeting helps!

Other safety measures include:

➤ Skate with a partner. Just in case something happens, there's a person right there to help provide first aid and get emergency help.

➤ Note the locations of public phones in case of emergency.

➤ Wear bright colors.

➤ Skate during the day.

➤ Find a locale where car traffic is light—or, better yet, where there is no traffic at all. A park is best.

➤ Notice the landscape around you—and avoiding oil slicks, rocks and pebbles, and glass.

The most common injury during inline skating is a broken wrist as a result of a fall. See Chapter 21 to learn about first aid for broken bones.

Ice Queens and Kings

Ice skating is the fastest growing spectator sport in America, thanks in part to the Nancy Kerrigan/Tonya Harding debacle in the Winter Olympics of 1994.

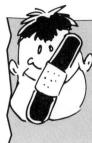

Before You Put the Band-Aid On

The televised broadcast of woman's figure skating in the Winter Olympics of 1994 was the most watched event in the history of sports broadcasting. The drama escalated when Nancy Kerrigan, who came in second, complained on camera about the gold medalist's tears of joy.

If you have the urge to leave the couch and join in the fun, there are some ground rules you should follow for safety's sake:

➤ Get a few lessons under your belt before attempting to go on the ice.

➤ Purchase or rent skates that fit. Skates should fit snugly, but your toes should not press against the tip. Try on skates with the socks you'll be wearing.

➤ Lacing of skates is crucial. They must be tight to keep ankles straight, but they should not cut off your circulation. It can take up to ten minutes to tie your skates properly, but it's worth it!

➤ Wear two or three layers of cotton socks under your skates. You don't want your feet to get numb from the cold.

➤ Avoid blisters by making sure your skates fit comfortably and have a slight bit of room at the toe, even with your socks on. (See Chapter 18 for treatment of blisters.)

➤ If you have weak ankles or flat feet, it might be difficult to ice skate. If your feet start to ache halfway around the arena, you might want to try a different sport.

➤ Wear breathable clothing that won't interfere with your skates; tights or stretch pants are best.

Ice skating doesn't have the same safety rules as inline skating. You don't need a helmet or knee pads because you'll rarely get up to fast speeds unless you are at the professional level. However, knee pads are not a bad idea for children and beginners, who are going to fall at least once, no doubt!

The most common ice-skating accidents come from falls. They include broken or sprained wrists and bruised bottoms (not to mention wounded pride). See Chapter 4 for emergency first aid treatment.

The Least You Need to Know

➤ Golf injuries occur most often as a result of improper golf swing techniques.

➤ Avoid heat prostration by carrying and using a water bottle and by keeping active sports to the early morning or early evening hours.

➤ "Tennis elbow" is an inflammation around the bony knob on the outside of the elbow. It is caused by poor shock absorption during serves and backhand swings.

➤ Wear proper safety equipment when you go inline skating, especially a helmet and wrist guards.

➤ Get at least one professional lesson before heading out on ice skates. Your body will thank you for it!

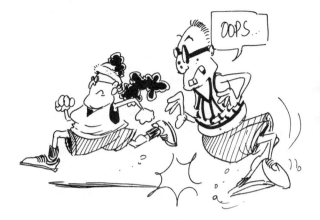

Chapter 33

Jogging, Swimming, and Other Exercise Injuries

In This Chapter

➤ Walking the correct way and avoiding injury

➤ The most common swimmer's injury

➤ Discovering the best aerobic class for you

➤ How to make the most of your exercise machine

➤ Which is safer: a stationary bike or an outdoor bike?

It's been imprinted on our minds. Exercise is healthy. Exercise to feel great. Exercise to lose weight. Exercise to reduce stress. Exercise to keep from aging.

But how do you know if you're doing the right exercises and if you're doing them properly? And, most importantly, how can you perform your exercise routine safely and avoid injury?

Exercise is good for you. No doubt about it. And by choosing a regimen you can enjoy, you'll be assured of sticking with it. Add the fact that you're taking safety precautions to avoid injury, and you'll stay motivated for life!

Exercise Choice 1: Jogging and Walking

Walking is considered one of the safest exercises around. Anyone, at any age, and at any fitness level, can do it. There's no special equipment (except sturdy shoes) and no special technique. Just put on a pair of walking shoes and go!

It's a fact. Walking is easy and fun. There's very little chance of injury unless you push too hard or don't follow basic safety measures.

Pushing too hard is easy when you're walking. After all, you've been doing it your entire life! Besides, there you are, enjoying the spring day with your Walkman playing some fast music. Why not go faster and further …until …ouch! Your heart begins to beat too fast, your leg cramps, and you can't catch your breath.

To avoid problems when you are walking or jogging, stay in your target heart rate zone.

Target Your Heart Rate

Your heart beats a specific number of times each minute. With every beat, or contraction, oxygen-rich blood is pushed out through your body. The more per minute beats, the more oxygen your muscles are receiving from the blood—which translates into a higher metabolism, more energy, and greater fitness potential.

Before you can determine your target heart rate, first determine your maximum heart rate (MHR). Subtract your age from 220 to find your MHR. (For example, if you are 20 years old, your MHR is 220–20 = 200.)

After you've determined your MHR, you can figure out your target zone which is the best pace (beats per minute) you can set for maximum benefits and minimum health risk.

Fifty to 60 percent of your MHR is considered the best place to start if you've never exercised before. Using our 20-year-old as an example, her target heart rate zone would be between 100–120 beats per minute.

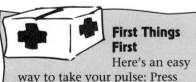

First Things First

Here's an easy way to take your pulse: Press two fingers on the inside of your wrist, the inside of your neck, or at your temple. As soon as you feel a beat, look at your watch and count the beats for 15 seconds and then multiply that number by four.

Seventy to 80 percent is best if you've already been exercising, but what if you still prefer the couch to the great outdoors? If you were our 20-year-old, you'd leave your MTV and go out for a walk or a jog that would give you a target heart rate zone between 140–170 beats per minute.

If target heart rate zones sound too complicated, use a "perceived rate of exertion" instead. It's easy. If you can still carry on a conversation, but you feel your heart pumping away, you are at the place you should be. If your walk or jog seems a bit too easy, pick up the pace. If you are having trouble catching your breath, slow down.

And always start your walk or jog with a warm up and some stretches. Finish with a cool down (a slow walk home).

Safety Measures and First Aid Treatment

Walking is practically injury-free. The only problems you might incur include corns, calluses, strains, and sprains. The occasional corn or callus can be taken care of with over-the-counter medications. However, if calluses hurt so much that they prevent you from walking comfortably, see a podiatrist. Strains and sprains are more common among joggers than walkers. The tendon that runs from the calf to the foot is the most common trouble spot. See Chapter 21, "Muscle Cramps, Strains, Sprains, and Breaks," for details on treating such injuries.

Here are some tips you can follow to prevent injury:

➤ Walk or jog in your target heart rate zone

➤ Walk or run with a buddy

➤ Vary your path and routine

➤ Exercise in the daytime for safety's sake. You'll also be seen by cars and bicycles!

➤ Avoid traffic-congested streets

➤ Carry a water bottle, and drink plenty of liquid

➤ Dress in layers in cold weather. When you get warm, you can peel off a layer and tie it around your waist without missing a beat.

➤ Wear loose clothing in hot weather.

➤ Walk in an air-conditioned mall if the weather is over 90 degrees.

➤ Make sure you warm up and stretch before beginning your walk or jog. This keeps muscles supple and flexible.

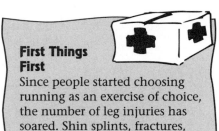

First Things First
Since people started choosing running as an exercise of choice, the number of leg injuries has soared. Shin splints, fractures, and tendonitis are common among enthusiastic beginners who leap too far too fast.

Exercise Choice 2: Swimming

Swimming (without sharks) is a good exercise for anyone who is recovering from a sports injury. The water keeps your body buoyant and there's no danger of impact. But there are a few things to remember to prevent injuries during swimming:

➤ Wear well-fitting goggles. Exposure to chlorine can burn your eyes. Goggles that are too tight can cause pressure to build up between your eyes and the lens—resulting in a black eye!

➤ Put some conditioner in your hair before taking the plunge. The harsh chemicals in the pool can harm hair follicles; the conditioner acts like an "invisible bathing cap."

➤ Avoid swimmer's shoulder. The repetitive motion of arm over head causes irritation in the shoulder, even though you're in water. The best advice is to start slow. Tread water for five minutes before beginning your swim. Use gentle upward motions, and the moment you feel a cramp, stop for the day.

➤ Listen to your body. If you start getting "goose bumps" and your lips are turning blue, it's time to stop. You might not freeze to death, but you could be ripe for an attack of cold or flu germs. Keep a towel nearby to wrap around you as soon as you get out of the water.

Exercise Choice 3: Aerobics Classes

Ten years ago, aerobics classes were all the rage. You could walk into any gym and hear the music blasting, the feet stomping, and the instructor screaming. Today, we know better. The motto for aerobics is no longer "No pain, no gain." Instead, the refrain of the '90s is "Go slow."

Low-impact classes have taken the place of high-impact classes. The difference? High-impact workouts include moves and jumps that take both feet off the floor. Low-impact aerobics, on the other hand, use moves in which one foot remains on the floor at all times—which means less stress and less risk of injury.

The following list gives you some safety tips to follow when you're doing aerobics:

➤ Go at your own pace. Even if the rest of the class is leaping four feet in the air, stay put if you feel you're overexerting yourself. You don't have to be a champion your first class. Follow your heart—your target heart rate zone, that is.

➤ Drink water. Slip out of class to use the water fountain if you need a drink. Don't wait for the class to stop. You might be dehydrated by then.

➤ Wear comfortable clothing. Wearing properly fitting sports bras, easy fitting leotards, non-tugging jock straps, and shorts that stay put, can all make a class more pleasurable (instead of an uncomfortable torture).

➤ Get the right pair of shoes. Walking shoes just aren't going to work for an aerobics class. Ditto tennis shoes. The wrong shoe can translate into sprains and cramps. If you want to avoid having a closet full of sports shoes, opt for a pair of cross-trainers. Try them on with socks. Make sure they offer support without being too tight.

Exercise Choice 4: Exercise Machines

We now know that aerobic exercise must be combined with a program of strength-training exercise for maximum cardiac health (and better weight loss, too!) One burns calories, the other increases lean muscle tissue. That's where exercise machines come in. The strange apparatus that stands in your gym or glares out from the latest TV infomercial helps build resistance and turn fat tissue into muscle tissue.

The best way to find the right exercise machine for you is to try as many as you can. Go to an exercise equipment store in the mall and try out their machines. Join a local health club and get some professional advice from a trainer. The best strength-training exercise regime incorporates a variety of machines to use different muscle groups. Weights should be easy to add or remove so that you can make sure you're working with the amount that's right for you. Free hand weights are also used for strengthening muscles. Several good videos are available that teach proper technique and safety. A good one to try is Kathy Smith's *Workout with Weights*.

Other exercise machines that work up a sweat include stationary bikes, stair climbers, skiing machines, and treadmills. These machines can be used for an aerobic workout, but they shouldn't be confused with the weight-bearing machines that strengthen and tone.

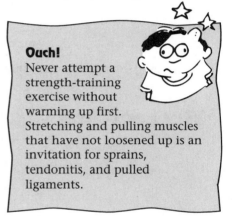

Ouch!
Never attempt a strength-training exercise without warming up first. Stretching and pulling muscles that have not loosened up is an invitation for sprains, tendonitis, and pulled ligaments.

Exercise Choice 5: Bicycling

It's all a matter of choice. Some people like the interior of a gym and a LifeCycle to pedal. Others like the great outdoors—the hills and valleys and the sound of the birds. Either way, indoors or out, you can get a good aerobic workout. But there are some safety precautions you should take and some first aid steps you'll need to know in an emergency.

One injury that's common among bicyclists is a broken collarbone (because of the position of the upper torso). See Chapter 21 for step-by-step first aid instructions for treating broken bones, strains, and sprains. Other injuries are dangers that arise if you fall off. See Chapter 16 for information on treating head injuries. Minor discomforts such as hemorrhoids can occur when you sit for a long time. To learn about finding relief, look to Chapter 27.

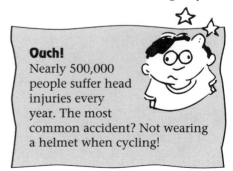

Ouch!
Nearly 500,000 people suffer head injuries every year. The most common accident? Not wearing a helmet when cycling!

Indoor cycling is not dangerous, as long as you don't push too hard. Outdoor cycling, however, requires more safety precautions:

➤ Always wear a helmet.

➤ Choose your outdoor bike carefully. Mountain bikes are more stable than road bicycles, even for city roads. They are a good choice for novice riders.

➤ Add reflective gear and lights if you are planning to ride at dusk or at night.

➤ Ride your bike in less congested areas.

➤ Bicycle with a friend.

➤ Use a thick band to tie pants legs close to the body. This way they won't accidentally get caught in the spokes of the wheel.

➤ Carry a plastic water bottle. You can purchase one that fits on the bicycle frame.

➤ Test your tires and brakes before beginning your ride.

The Least You Need to Know

➤ Combine aerobic exercise with strength-training exercise.

➤ Use the right shoe for the right exercise, or opt for a cross-trainer.

➤ Exercise in your target heart rate zone, and always warm up.

➤ Alternate your aerobic activities: walk one day, bicycle the next, swim the third.

➤ Avoid high-impact aerobics unless you're extremely fit. Low-impact classes do the job just fine.

➤ Always wear a helmet when you ride a bicycle.

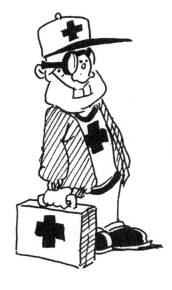

Aid for All Seasons

You might plan your vacations according to the season, but medical emergencies know nothing about the weather. Injuries can occur anytime, whether you're in Brussels, Rome, Mexico, or right at home.

Traveling in any season can be a joy—or a burden. Do your homework before you go. Know what to expect. And plan, plan, plan. That way, all you have to do when you arrive is have fun!

In the Good Old Summertime

Barbecues, swimming, piling cool sand on your feet, feeling the sun on your face... finding a party of ants in your picnic basket, ending a day at the beach with a lobster-red face, getting a bee sting ...these are the joys and the dangers of summer.

But the dangers can be nothing more than unpleasant memories if you take a few precautions:

➤ Use sunscreen when in the sun, and reapply frequently, especially after swimming.

➤ Drink plenty of water to avoid dehydration.

➤ Avoid the sun between ten in the morning and two in the afternoon.

➤ Wear waterproof sandals to avoid bites and pebble pain.

➤ Avoid swimming if there's a school of jellyfish in sight.

➤ Use insect repellent to keep the bugs away.

Sailing, Sailing

Unfortunately, not everyone observes boating safety rules. All a person needs is a driver's license (which isn't even mandatory in some states!), and he or she can rev up the engine, drink and drive, and generally create havoc until the Coast Guard or other patrol orders him or her to stop.

But, not every problem is caused by someone else. Here are some precautions you can take to make sure that boating remains pleasure:

➤ Always wear a life jacket, even if you are an Olympic swimmer.

➤ If a person happens to fall overboard, his or her life jacket should help. However, you should stop your boat and throw a life preserver out into the water to help "pull" the overboard person in. Radio for help, if you have a radio (and you should have one for safety's sake!). Get the person back in the boat and check for injuries that may require medical attention.

➤ Pay attention to the weather. You don't want to be caught in a storm when you're out in a boat.

Fishing First Aid

If the fishhook you plan to throw in the water gets caught in someone's skin instead, don't panic. Follow these steps for quick first aid:

1. If the point is the only part of the hook in the skin, gently pull it out.

2. If the barb is embedded in the skin, wait for help to arrive, if you've radioed ahead and are in a high-traffic area. But if you are in the middle of an isolated lake, cut the line and get to shore to seek help.

3. Do not try to remove a fishhook that's embedded in the face.

4. *Never* pull out a barbed fishhook the way it went in. In fact, if possible, wait for a health professional to do the job. It will decrease the chance of infection! But if no one is around and the hook is near the surface of the skin, gently push it through to the other side. Cut the barb off so you can safely pull the hook out.

5. Makes sure you follow first aid precautions for treating wounds and cuts (see Chapter 3).

6. Always seek medical help, taking care to consider the risk of tetanus.

First Things First
A boater's first aid kit looks just like a landlubber's kit, except for a few items such as an inflatable float, sturdy rope, a magnifying glass for removing jellyfish stingers, and a waterproof container to hold fishhooks, fish, and tentacles that you've removed and need to show to a health professional.

Foreign Travel

When you travel, don't forget to take your prescription medications. Some countries don't have medication available, and other countries, such as Europe, have different medications than those in the United States. You might have trouble finding the medication you need.

If you're traveling in southern Europe, in Italy, Portugal, or Greece, drink bottled water. And, although it sounds ridiculous, take a roll of toilet paper from home. The European type is much more harsh.

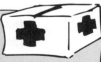

First Things First
If you're planning a trip to Scandinavia in the summer, don't forget to add a sweater or two. The weather is always cooler in the Northern climes. And be prepared for longer starry nights.

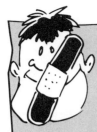

Before You Put the Band-Aid On

If you're going to Mexico or South America, make sure to take along your water! To avoid "Montezuma's Revenge" (described in Chapter 27), use bottled water for drinking, brushing your teeth, and washing your face. Do not eat salad or anything else that might have been washed in foreign water, and avoid drinks with ice cubes.

You'll also need certain vaccines, such as a yellow fever vaccine. Make sure you take prophylactic medication if you are going to areas where malaria is a possibility. Check with the passport office.

Winter Wonderland

Snow can be beautiful—especially if you don't have to shovel it! All those soft white flakes waiting for you to ski down. Or the frozen lake, waiting for you to skate. Yes, winter has its own charms and pleasures. To enjoy them safely, remember some safety tips:

➤ Avoid frostbite by dressing in layers on the slope. (See Chapter 18 for treating frostbite.)

➤ Wear sunglasses and sunscreen in ski country. The sun on the snow can be as blinding and dangerous as the summer sun.

➤ Before skating on a frozen lake or pond, make sure the ice is thick enough to hold your weight. In addition, check to see if there are any warnings posted.

➤ A fall into ice cold water can cause hypothermia. If that happens, get help as soon as possible. (See Chapter 10 for more information on drowning and Chapter 18 for more on hypothermia.)

Spring Ahead, Fall Behind

Spring and fall provide the perfect conditions for camping, hiking, and exploring. It's warm enough to enjoy the outdoors, but cool enough to keep insects away. To ensure good health, here's some advice:

➤ Spring is allergy time. Make sure you've had your shots or take your medication with you.

➤ Keep asthma inhalers in your first aid kit. (See Chapter 7 for instructions for treating asthma attacks.)

➤ Dress appropriately. It might feel warm, but your body has yet to adjust to warmer/ cooler temperatures. To ward off colds and flu in the spring or fall, wear a light parka or sweater. A scarf at the neck also keeps chills away. Always dress in layers that can be removed as you get warmer or added when the temperature drops).

➤ Avoid nasty insects and poisonous plants such as ticks, mosquitoes, poison ivy, and poison oak. Wear long pants, socks, long-sleeved shirts, and hats—especially if you're hiking in the woods.

Camping

From hiking in the woods to climbing rocks, camping is a nature lover's dream—or nightmare, if you're not prepared. Before you go camping, ask yourself these questions:

1. Where are you going? Will it be hot or cold? Make sure you take the right clothes.

2. Who is going? How many people? Take plenty of food and diversions, as well as any necessary medications and allergy provisions.

3. How far are you going to take "roughing it?" Remember who your family is—and who you really are. If you're on your first camping trip, don't attempt Mount Everest. Stay in a clean, well-lighted, registered campsite.

4. What emergencies can come up? Will you face snakes? Possible rock slides? Spiders?

5. What do you want to get out of this vacation? Relaxation or an outward bound experience? Pack your first aid kit accordingly! (See information on portable first aid kits later in this chapter.)

6. Always leave a detailed itinerary with someone you trust who is staying behind. Never head off alone!

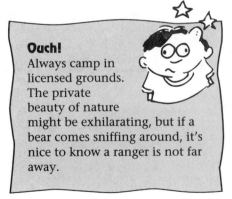

Ouch!
Always camp in licensed grounds. The private beauty of nature might be exhilarating, but if a bear comes sniffing around, it's nice to know a ranger is not far away.

First Aid Kits for Outdoor Adventurers

Some prepackaged first aid kits are better than others. Here are some near-perfect prepackaged kits that are available:

The Walkabout First Aid Kit from Atwater and Carey. In addition to the usual first aid accouterments, you'll also find pill vials, sting-relief pads, antibiotics, and antihistamines (Benadryl). The nylon case has plenty of room for extras you might want to take along.

Johnson & Johnson's First Aid Kit. This plastic, lightweight kit holds every type of bandage and gauze you'll ever need. And there's room to add your own individual supplies.

Johnson & Johnson's Compact First Aid Kit. When room is a luxury, consider the compact version. It has almost everything that the larger size has, but fewer of each item.

Healer Products First Aid Kits. These lightweight, plastic kits contain just about everything you'll need in any emergency, including a superb antiseptic burn spray and an instant ice pack. These kits also come in various sizes.

And you might want to consider adding these items to the basics in any kit:

The "Snoozle." An inflatable pillow you can use anytime, anywhere, from airplanes to tents. They are especially useful if someone gets sick with the flu or a fever and needs to lie down comfortably.

Skeeter Beeters from TravelSmith. These nylon mesh pullover pants, tops, and hoods have elastic at the opening to make a perfect mosquito netting without the bed!

An emergency thermal blanket. REI makes one such blanket, which is a thin sheet of insulating material similar to those created for the Apollo space mission. It folds easily, and it actually works to keep you warm. It's especially good for hypothermia emergencies.

The Least You Need to Know

➤ Be careful and try to prevent sunburn and insects at the beach.

➤ Don't go skating on *any* ice unless you get official clearance.

➤ Always pack allergy medication and an inhaler if there's an asthmatic in the family.

➤ A prepackaged kit is fine—as long as you know how to customize it to meet your needs.

➤ Traveling abroad is exhilarating, but don't forget the essentials: your medication, bottled water, and toilet paper!

➤ Ask yourself the "six camping questions" before you drive off to any campground.

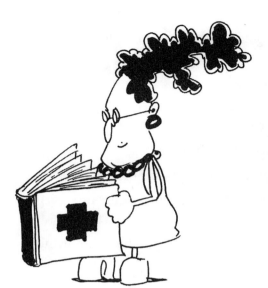

Glossary of First Aid

ABCs of First Aid   If you can remember these ABCs in the correct order, you can save a life. Make sure that Airways are open, Breathing is restored, and Circulation is maintained. In other words, check a person's breathing and pulse and take immediate first aid measures if anything is awry.

Ace bandage   An elastic strip of material that wraps and is secured with hooks around a sprained limb to keep the injury secure.

acute asthma   Associated with shortness of breath accompanied by wheezing. During an attack, the bronchial tubes constrict, impairing the flow of air into the lungs.

airway bag   An apparatus that facilitates "breathing" into another person's lungs while providing a sterile environment between you and the victim during mouth-to-mouth resuscitation.

anaphylactic reaction   An allergic reaction, usually to bee stings, in which the throat literally swells up so much that a person eventually won't be able to breathe. A prescription antihistamine and epinephrine must be administered immediately to neutralize the reaction.

antibiotic   A by-prescription-only medication that fights the bacteria and germs that lead to ear infections, body infections, bronchitis, and strep throat.

antihistamine   An over-the-counter pill, such as Benadryl, that stops the sneezing and sniffling of an allergy attack.

brainstem   The lower area of the brain that regulates breathing, the body's thermostat, and other bodily functions.

cardiac arrest   The heart suddenly stops beating.

Cardiopulmonary Resuscitation (CPR)   A special rhythmic resuscitation technique used when the heart stops beating. Training is required to do CPR correctly.

carotid artery   The large artery found on either side of the neck.

cerebellum   The area of the brain responsible for balance, among other things.

cerebrum   The area of the brain that holds our "higher functions," including speech, thought, logic, perception, and organizational skills.

concussion   Literally, a bang on the head. Although an outside wound can sometimes show, most of the damage is done inside, where the brain hits the skull. Most concussions are minor, clearing up after a few days of rest.

dysplasia   Abnormal tissue growth that can lead to cancer.

Emergency Medical Technician (EMT)   A trained professional who comes in the fully supplied ambulance when you call for help.

frostbite   A condition in which parts of the body "freeze" and are left without circulation. Frostbite is characterized by red and then gray-colored skin, which eventually turns a bright, icy color (the signal of tissue damage).

glaucoma   A condition in which fluid builds up in the eye. Ultimately, this pressure pushes on the optic nerve in the back of the eye and causes blindness.

gout   A condition caused by a build up of too much uric acid within the body. The uric acid creates crystals, which are deposited in the joints, making them swell and eventually "push" against nerve endings.

heat prostration   A condition that occurs from too much sun and dehydration. Symptoms include a temperature over 104 degrees Fahrenheit and profuse sweating. (In the elderly, heat prostration occurs when the body temperature reaches 100–102 degrees Fahrenheit.)

Heimlich Maneuver   A technique used to dislodge whatever is causing a person to choke. Named after its inventor, U.S. surgeon Henry J. Heimlich, this maneuver literally pushes out the food or object that is causing breathing problems. It involves applying sudden pressure with your fist, using an inward and upward thrust to the upper abdomen, to force the obstruction out.

hemorrhage   Excessive bleeding.

hyperventilation   A condition of rapid, over-breathing that occurs in acute anxiety attacks. Symptoms of the anxiety attack include numbness in the hands, feet, and mouth, a tingling sensation in the fingers and toes, an overwhelming feeling of panic, and an inability to catch one's breath.

ice compress   A cloth wrapped over ice or a chemically cold, flexible packet that is put on bumps, bruises, and sprains to reduce swelling.

immobilize   To keep an injured person completely still (especially used when a head or back injury is suspected). Immobilization can be achieved by using pillows as a brace and belts as straps. The victim may or may not be conscious and confused.

jellyfish   Gelatinous, cloudy-looking marine life whose tentacles hold a poison and a vicious sting.

limbic system   The area of the brain most responsible for our emotions.

lobe   One of several sections or areas of the brain where different functions are controlled. For example, the frontal lobe, near the forehead, holds our "higher" functions, the parts of us that make us human and uniquely us.

maximum heart rate (MHR)   The most times within a minute that your heart should beat, given your particular age.

Medic Alert   A bracelet or necklace that is made by a company in California. On one side is the Medic Alert symbol: a staff and a snake. The other side contains vital information about the person wearing it: allergies, diabetes, or epilepsy. It also gives a phone number that someone can call to receive a more complete medical history. Medic Alert bracelets can mean the difference between life and death if someone is unconscious.

menopause   A condition in women in their forties and fifties when the estrogen levels in their bodies begin to drop. Perimenopause is the period leading up to menopause.

mouth-to-mouth resuscitation   A technique used if a person has stopped breathing. Holding the neck up with one hand and pinching the nose with the other, you take a deep breath, then exhale directly into the victim's mouth. Wait a few seconds, then repeat.

neurologist   A medical doctor who specializes in diseases and conditions of the nervous system, including head injury, brain tumors, spinal cord injury, and concussion.

neuron   Another name for the nerve cells found in the brain.

obstetrician   A physician trained to treat pregnant women from conception to birth.

ophthalmologist   A medical doctor who specializes in diseases of the eye. He or she is trained to not only examine eyes, but also diagnose and treat various conditions of the eye, such as cataracts and glaucoma.

Post-Concussion Syndrome A condition where neurological capabilities and psychological emotions can deteriorate slowly over time.

Premenstrual Syndrome (PMS) A very real physical reaction to the changes in hormonal structure that occur two weeks before menstruation. Besides mood change and water retention, this hormonal change also leads to the blood vessel constriction that causes cramps.

pulse The movement of the blood through your arteries. At each heart beat, the walls of the arteries swell with blood. Between beats, as the blood moves along, the walls shrink back to normal size. The rhythmic swelling and shrinking is what you feel when you take a person's pulse—at your inner wrist, at the side of your neck, and at your temple.

shock A condition in which the body's chemistry suddenly, immediately, and rapidly, goes out of whack. Symptoms include erratic breathing, clammy, pale skin, chills and nausea, weakness, and unconsciousness.

sitz bath A soak in a shallow-filled tub of warm water and baking soda. It is soothing for children with fever and women with yeast and urinary tract infections.

sling A triangular-shaped brace used to keep broken arms immobile and secured.

spiral technique A bandaging technique used to wrap knees and upper legs securely.

splint A device used to support and immobilize broken bones, fractures, sprains, and painful joints. A splint is any hard, straight object that is bandaged to the limb in question.

stroke A sudden disruption of the blood supply to a part of the brain, which, in turn, disrupts the body function controlled by that brain area (definition from The National Stroke Association).

syncope The official term for fainting, which means a temporary loss of consciousness due to a sudden, insufficient amount of blood flow to the brain.

Syrup of Ipecac A liquid that induces vomiting in case of poisoning.

Tetanus An infection, also known as "lockjaw," that literally paralyzes its victims.

tourniquet A device used when bleeding is so heavy that finger pressure doesn't stop it. A tourniquet can be anything from a belt to a shirt that is tied tightly a few inches above the cut to stop blood flow. Always check the tourniquet, however. It should be tight, but not tight enough to stop all circulation.

Universal Guidelines New official rules and regulations that hospital staff, physicians, and health professionals must follow in order to prevent transmission of disease or highly infectious viruses such as HIV. An example of a universal guideline is to always wear latex gloves when treating a patient.

Index

339

N-O

P

T